Dear Reader,
Thank you for buying my book!
I want to say *Thank you!*
Here is a little gift from me/

You can try your luck in a ***Grand Amazon Raffle*** (the biggest prize is – **95% discount** for a travel toiletry bag) and also you can win 5$ gift card in a lottery!

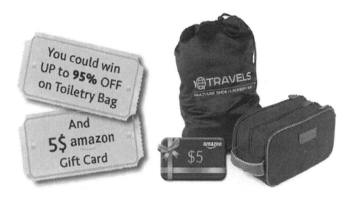

More under this QR – code

Or just type this link:
https://www.facebook.com/iqtravelsUsa/posts/1970842956516913

Contents

Chapter 1: Discovering FODMAPs and How They Affect Your Digestive Health

Introduction

It is estimated that somewhere between ten and fifteen percent of the world's population suffers from the symptoms of Irritable Bowel Syndrome, more commonly referred to as IBS. The symptoms of this condition range from bloating and gas to disruptive changes in bowel habits and severe abdominal pain. While the exact cause of IBS in individuals is not known, it is a generally well accepted theory that diet and food sensitivities play a major role in gastrointestinal conditions and how the symptoms present themselves.

For years, people who suffered with these symptoms struggled on their own while attempting to identify the foods that triggered their individual symptoms. Then, in 2005, a group of researchers from Monash University in Australia discovered that when certain foods, now known as FODMAPs, were eliminated from the diets of IBS sufferers, that approximately seventy-five percent of them had a reduction in overall symptoms.

While the scientific research about the use of low-FODMAP foods has been primarily centered around the treatment of IBS, for this book, I would also like to include those who suffer from other types of Functional Gastrointestinal Disorders (FGIDs) such as, functional dyspepsia, abdominal migraine, functional constipation and cyclic vomiting syndrome, among others. While research is limited in the use of FODMAPs in treating FGIDs, there is promising potential that low-FODMAP foods can help to ease symptoms from a variety of conditions in addition to IBS. Some people with food sensitivities such as celiac disease and irritable bowel syndrome might be able to find some relief as well although they should consult with their doctor before embarking on this or any other eating plan.

FODMAP is an acronym for Fermentable Oligosaccharides, Disaccharides, Monosaccharides and Polyols. This group of saccharides and polyols are short-chain carbohydrates that can cause havoc in your gut. The FODMAP diet is essentially an elimination plan that removes potential digestive triggers from your daily diet. While the elimination of dietary triggers is important for long term health, the FODMAP diet is one that is followed for only a few weeks at a time. Our plan is one that is designed as a four-week program. Then, one at a time, individual types of eliminated foods are slowly reintroduced, giving you an opportunity to notice how each type of food affects you personally, so that you can permanently eliminate the foods that cause you painful digestive distress and adjust your daily diet as needed.

The FODMAP acronym stands for some big words that you don't often find on nutritional labels, so how do you go about knowing which foods are high FODMAP (bad) foods and which one are low FODMAP (good) foods? While avoiding sugary and processed foods is important for your health, no matter what diet you follow, the FODMAP plan goes further to recognize foods that can disrupt gut health, but that are otherwise generally nutritious. For example, onions, garlic, apples, lactose containing dairy products and legumes are all high FODMAP foods which may contribute to your intestinal distress. Some of these foods might be your triggers while you may find that others are safe for you to enjoy in limited or moderate quantities.

Most people tend to associate the word "diet" with a meal plan that is restrictive, in one way or another, for the purpose of losing weight with trend diets coming and going quickly. While the FODMAP diet has been becoming more recognized lately, it is important to say that the purpose of this diet is not to lose weight, or even eat "healthier." The FODMAP diet is an eating plan that is designed to be therapeutic, to ease symptoms of painful digestive disease and to increase your quality of life.

The FODMAP diet is both scientifically proven and internationally accepted as a method of controlling the symptoms of IBS and other digestive disorders. The common symptoms of IBS include nausea, pain, bloating, flatulence, vomiting and changes in bowel habits. However, what goes on in the gut has an overwhelming effect on the rest of the body and people with IBS symptoms also sometimes suffer from unexpected symptoms such as fatigue, depression and poor concentration, just to name a few.

The FODMAP diet is a healing plan that helps you relearn how to properly and effectively nourish your body while reducing the uncomfortable, painful and sometimes embarrassing symptoms of digestive distress. You could be just a few weeks away from enjoying the freedom that comes from having control over your digestive health.

Breaking Apart the Acronym
When we break apart the acronym for FODMAP, we are left with some sizable words that you probably don't run across every day. You certainly won't find most of them on your food labels, so how do you know which foods meet the FODMAP criteria and which ones don't? It all starts with understanding the components. Let's begin breaking it down.

- Fermentable: In relation to the FODMAP diet, fermentable refers to a group of carbohydrates that are easily fermented in your digestive system, primarily in the large intestines. This type of fermentation plays a major role in the development of IBS symptoms such as bloating, gas, pain and changes in bowel patterns.

- Oligosaccharide: Called "oligos" for short, this is a saccharide polymer, usually composed of somewhere between two and ten sugar molecules, which bond together and form a chain. Two of the most common oligos that ferment in the digestive system are fructans and galacto-oligosaccharides, also called GOS. These carbohydrates are problematic because our bodies lack the ability to break down these chains into simple sugars which can be absorbed. Since we can't absorb them, it means that they stick around in the intestinal lining where they quickly ferment.

- Disaccharide: The prefix "di" means two, and the word saccharide, which you will be seeing quite a bit in this book, is the word for a sugar molecule. Just as oligosaccharide indicates multiple sugar molecules, a disaccharide is composed of two sugar molecules. While you are probably familiar with different types of disaccharides such as simple table sugar or sucrose, it is the disaccharide lactose that is the most problematic for IBS sufferers. Lactose is a sugar molecule, formed by glucose and galactose, that is naturally occurring in milk and dairy products.

- Monosaccharide: Monosaccharides are single carbohydrate molecules often referred to as simple sugars. Fructose is the monosaccharide of the most concern in the FODMAP diet. Not everyone has difficulty absorbing fructose, so not everyone will be sensitive to this particular carbohydrate. Fructose is naturally occurring in many fresh, nutritious fruits. However, that does not mean that you need to eliminate all those fruits from your diet. How fructose is paired up with other carbohydrates, such as glucose, significantly impacts how easily the sugar is broken down and absorbed.

- Polyols: These are sugar alcohol molecules, but not the kind that can leave you with a bad headache the next day from overconsumption. However, polyols can leave you with a bad gut ache if you are not careful. You are probably most familiar with polyols under their more common names of Erythritol, Isomalt, Maltitol, Sorbitol and Xylitol. If you don't recognize any of these names, go look in your pantry and read your food labels, chances are that you will find one of these names of sugar substitutes at least once. Polyols add the taste and texture of sugar, without the added calories. These types of sugar alcohols are only partially digested in the intestines, providing lots of food for the fermentation process.

While it is important to be able to recognize the trigger foods that are part of the FODMAP plan, it is equally important to acknowledge that these foods are not the cause of IBS, FGIDs or other digestive disorders; rather these foods promote certain symptoms within your body, symptoms of a condition, or intolerance, that still exists with or without these foods. The foods cause the symptoms, but not the condition itself. This is the reason behind the process of eliminating and reintroducing each group of foods. Some people will have sensitivities to all components of the FODMAPs while others will only be sensitive to a few, and possibly only one. Eliminating these foods will not cure your sensitivity or intolerance, but without these foods in your diet, your body cannot react to them, and through that your symptoms can be relieved.

Feeling the Fermentation

As you looked at the FODMAP groups listed above, did you notice a common theme? If you picked up on the word "fermentation," then you have discovered the key to FODMAPs. Each of the FODMAP components causes distress as a direct result of malabsorption and the fermentation that follows.

During the course of this book, it might seem like fermentation is getting a bad reputation. The truth is that fermentation, on its own, isn't such a bad thing. In fact, the fermentation process produces food for the healthy bacteria in your gut that work so hard to keep everything running smoothly. The problem is that some of us are more sensitive to the effects of fermentation than others. For those who suffer from IBS or other digestive disorders, the fermentation process can be a double-edged sword. On one side you have bloating, pain and gas caused by the fermentation, and on the other side, you have the associated osmotic effect, which means more water is drawn into your bowels, resulting in diarrhea or an increase in bowel frequency.

To really understand how the elimination of FODMAPs can help you, it is beneficial to start with a solid understanding of the fermentation process and how it affects your digestive health.

Your digestive system is lined with billions of bacteria and other microorganisms. You have a population of bacteria in your gut that rivals, if not exceeds, the entire human population on earth. These bacteria are necessary. So necessary in fact, that it is suggested that many chronic diseases that affect all parts of the body are brought about by an imbalance of digestive microbes and an unhealthy digestive system. Just like you, these bacteria require fuel, in the form of food, to survive and do their job. This fuel comes from the unabsorbed molecules that hang around in your digestive system. As a byproduct of fermentation, hydrogen, methane and other gases are produced. It is these gases that expand the intestinal walls and cause the painful symptoms of IBS and digestive distress.

To put it in the most basic of terms, unabsorbed carbohydrates hang around in the intestines, basically becoming stuck to the intestinal walls. Here, they are exposed to bacteria which rapidly begin fermenting them, and as a result, natural byproducts are produced. For some reason, which is still unknown, people with IBS experience worse and more painful symptoms of this process. When we look at the FODMAP components, we recognize fermentation as the common factor, but the process of each is slightly different. Therefore, you might be sensitive to one type of FODMAP but not another.

For example, let's take a look at the oligos. As mentioned earlier, the FODMAP oligos category is composed of fructans and galacto-oligosaccharides. Fructans are chains of fructose molecules joined together with a glucose molecule attached at the end. To completely absorb fructans, the body needs to completely break down the molecule into single molecule sugars, or monosaccharides. The problem is that the body is not capable of this process. We simply do not naturally possess the enzymes necessary for this process. This is true regardless of whether you suffer from digestive disorders or not. Since, these molecules cannot be completely broken down and absorbed, they linger in the large intestine where they will come face to face with bacteria that are eager to begin the fermentation process. The other type of oligos, galacto-oligosaccharides, are also chains of sugar molecules with a glucose attached at the end. These molecules also cannot be absorbed because we lack the necessary enzymes to do so.

Next, we can take a look at the disaccharides, such as lactose, sucrose and maltose. Lactose is a molecule of glucose and galactose joined together. When you consume something that contains the lactose molecule, such as milk, ice cream and many other types of dairy, your body uses an enzyme called lactase to break it down. While we are capable of breaking down lactose, unlike the oligos which we do not have the capability to break down at all, some of us don't produce enough lactase to break it down completely. The result is lactose intolerance or a sensitivity associated with IBS and other digestive disorders. On the other hand, it is only in very rare situations that we have difficulty breaking down other disaccharides such as sucrose.

The monosaccharides, particularly fructose, are a problem for many people with IBS. In fact, it is estimated that approximately seventy percent of people with IBS have symptoms that are exaggerated by fructose. In a healthy digestive system, there are transporter proteins found within the intestines whose job it is to help the fructose molecule become absorbed and used for energy. However, it seems that some people, such as a majority of IBS sufferers, have transporter proteins that are dysfunctional and don't do their job properly. Therefore, the fructose molecules sit around waiting to be fermented in your gut.

The issue with fructose is of particular concern because there are actually many nutritious foods that contain fructose. Most fruits, some vegetables and honey all contain fructose. Do you need to forgo these naturally healthy foods for the sake of your digestive health? No, not all of them. How easily you can absorb fructose depends not only on the transporter proteins in the gut, but also the amount of glucose that accompanies the fructose molecule. When glucose is present, in amounts that are equal to or greater than the amount of fructose present, the fructose molecule can attach itself to the glucose, and basically piggy back its way through the intestinal wall, even without properly functioning transporter proteins. Therefore, you might notice that some fructose containing foods are on the high FODMAP list, while others are on the low FODMAP list. It all depends on what the fructose is partnered with.

Then, we come to the polyols, which in most cases can be absorbed, the problem being that they are simply absorbed too slowly. Because these molecules take so long to be absorbed along the intestinal lining, the fermentation process usually begins before absorption is complete. Along with this, even the polyols that did get absorbed are problematic because they have an osmotic effect, pulling water molecules into the intestines, causing or worsening already present symptoms of digestive distress.

So, now you can see that each of the FODMAPs causes digestive distress under slightly different circumstances, but each one relates back to the root cause of fermentation. The key to healing your digestive system lies in learning to recognize which of these types of carbohydrates cause you the most distress. Your symptoms might be due to an oversensitivity to the fermentation of oligos, or maybe you produce less lactase than the average person. Perhaps, you will discover that you suffer from difficulties with all the FODMAPs, but chances are you will learn that there are only a couple that really present a problem for your gut health. Unfortunately, there is not a simple test to discover your individual sensitivities to FODMAPs, so it therefore becomes necessary to make this discovery through other means, such as the FODMAP diet.

Within just four weeks you will experience less pain, less symptoms of IBS and FGID, more energy and an overall improved mindset and quality of life. Four weeks for all of that doesn't sound so bad, does it? Next, let's talk about whether the FODMAP plan is really right for you.

Chapter 2: Is the Low-FODMAP Diet Plan Right for You?

If you suffer from IBS and symptoms of chronic digestive distress, then you are likely all too aware that your food choices significantly impact the presence and severity of your symptoms. Before the FODMAP diet was discovered, narrowing down the foods that caused the worst symptoms was a complicated guessing game at best. Even today, many people still suffer unnecessarily from painful symptoms that can be eased with the correct knowledge. In fact, it is estimated that only ten percent of the people who suffer from symptoms of IBS actually seek medical help. This means that there is an incredible number of people out there, suffering quietly with painful digestive issues.

Even those of us who do seek help for our symptoms are often led down a path of nutritional advice that can be more harmful than healing. To be fair, the varied symptoms and severity of IBS can make it difficult to easily recognize and treat. For example, many people with IBS deal with chronic diarrhea or constipation. If you were to go to a doctor and describe just these symptoms, you might be told to add more soluble fiber to your diet. Soluble fiber is great, and beneficial to your health, unless you have IBS where certain forms of it can make your symptoms worse. Foods like apples and fiber fortified wheat breads are excellent sources of soluble fiber. They are also on the high-FODMAP food list. Essentially, the very foods that you are eating to ease your symptoms are only making them worse.

This is in part because as part of their education, doctors are taught to look for the simplest explanation first, because often, it is the correct diagnosis. In many cases, this is beneficial for both the doctor and the patient. Is it necessary to go through the process of and costs of sophisticated diagnostic tests if your issue can be easily addressed without going through all of that? This philosophy saves doctors and patients time and allows physicians to begin treatment faster. The problem is when the treatment doesn't work, and you go back looking for more answers.

For example, if you were told to add more soluble fiber to your diet, but not only does the addition not ease your symptoms but actually makes them worse, then it is time to look further, past the simple diagnosis to find the root cause of your distress. To further complicate matters, not all health care providers are fully informed on the physiological mechanisms involved with IBS, and therefore offer inadequate treatment plans. Many people with IBS symptoms become frustrated, or worse embarrassed, and stop seeking treatment after the initial suggestions don't work. If this is where you are on your journey, there is a good chance that the FODMAP diet can change your life.

There are theories on why some people suffer from the inability to absorb FODMAPS more than others. However, we still do not know the exact cause, especially since the potential causes seem to vary from person to person. It is thought that in some people there is an overgrowth of the bacteria found in the small intestine. This is referred to as SIBO (small intestine bacterial overgrowth). In a healthy gut, the bacteria population remains fairly stable, providing just the right amount to do the job effectively. For some people, this population grows and exceeds normal levels. Remember how we said that bacteria and other microbes really aren't all that different from us in how they need food to survive and function? In the case of an excessive microbial population, you have a large population that is hungry and looking for food, which may become a scarcity due to population size alone. So, as a survival mechanism, these overpopulated bacteria work faster and more ferociously to ferment FODMAP molecules before they even have the chance to potentially be absorbed.

Then there are those of us who lack the adequate enzymes to effectively breakdown and absorb the FODMAPs before they reach the colon. Additionally, it is suspected that our modern lifestyle can be partially to blame for the onset of the condition as well. Stress, particularly chronic stress, has been shown to disrupt the balance of gut flora, which essentially effects the way your body breaks down and absorbs nutrients. All of these possible causes are just that, "possible" answers. At this point, it simply isn't possible to detect the exact mechanism behind each individual's digestive symptoms, and because of that, you need an approach that first addresses all the potential triggers together and then gives you the opportunity to pinpoint your individual issues.

So, if high-FODMAP foods cause so much digestive distress, it is safe to assume that everyone can benefit from the FODMAP diet plan, right? The answer is that this statement isn't true at all. Most of the foods that are eliminated on a low-FODMAP eating plan are actually high in nutritive value. If you have a healthy digestive system, and these foods do not cause an increase in IBS and FGID symptoms, there is absolutely no reason to avoid them. In fact, it can be a detriment to your overall health to eliminate some of these foods if you do not have good reason for doing so.

This means that you must first decide if the FODMAP plan is your best option for relief. The first step to this is making an appointment to see your doctor. There is a blood test that your doctor can order that identifies anti-CdtB and anti-vinculin antibodies. These antibodies are typically elevated in people who suffer from IBS compared to the general population. This is a simple way to help diagnose IBS, but chances are that even with these tests, your doctor is going to look for specific symptomatic criteria, known as Rome III criteria, to make an official diagnosis.

To begin with, IBS is what is called a "ruled out" diagnosis. This means that other, simpler causes, need to be ruled out before the diagnosis is set. To meet the diagnostic criteria for IBS, a patient should exhibit the following:

Recurrent abdominal pain and/or discomfort at least three days per month for a period of at least three months plus at least two of the following three, additional criteria:

- Improvement of symptoms with defecation, present for the last three months with symptom onset at least six months prior to diagnosis
- Change of stool frequency, present for the last three months with symptom onset at least six months prior to diagnosis
- Change of stool form, present for the last three months with symptom onset at least six months prior to diagnosis

As you can see, the diagnosis of IBS is not one that is handed out to every patient who reports digestive distress, but rather to those patients who meet a detailed criteria outline. For this reason, it would be irresponsible of me to suggest that you self-diagnose and treat yourself for IBS. This diagnosis should always be made by a qualified physician. However, if you are experiencing frequent digestive symptoms, it is within your rights to treat those symptoms naturally and effectively as possible, including being aware of FODMAPs and how they affect your health.

If you experience only occasional digestive distress, the FODMAP elimination diet might not be for you. If your symptoms are occasional and minor, you might want to start off with a food journal, writing down everything that you eat and drink for a period of thirty to sixty days. When you eat processed foods, make sure to look at the food label and make note of any high-FODMAP ingredients. After a while, with an awareness of high and low-FODMAP foods, you might be able to narrow down the foods that are causing your occasional symptoms. At that point, you can then try a modified FODMAP program where you eliminate just those components that you have recognized as being bothersome.

However, if your digestive distress symptoms are more frequent and severe, it can be more difficult to identify your triggers through means other than dietary modifications. You might benefit from the FODMAP diet if you regularly experience the following symptoms:

- Recurrent abdominal pain
- Abdominal cramping
- Change in bowel habits
- Frequent diarrhea
- Frequent constipation
- Inability to completely empty the bowels
- Urgent need to empty the bowels
- Symptoms eased by emptying the bowels
- Excessive flatulence
- Indigestion

- Nausea
- Loss of appetite
- General bodily discomfort
- Depression
- Anxiety

If these symptoms sound like a rundown of your daily life, the chances are pretty good that you have more going on than a mild intolerance or indigestion. These symptoms are serious, they are significant and they can greatly impact your quality of life. Again, my advice is to contact a physician and talk about whether the FODMAP diet is right for you. With that, I can't deny that there is a large portion of sufferers who are unable or unwilling to receive medical care, and that each person deserves some relief from IBS and symptoms of digestive distress. If you find that you can answer yes, more than you answer no, to the list of symptoms, then you owe it to yourself to consider the low FODMAP eating plan. In a matter of just four weeks, you can relieve your symptoms and gain back control of your life with a plan that is scientifically proven to relieve your symptoms and is formulated to be nutritionally sound and well rounded

How do you know for sure that the low-FODMAP plan is right for you? Start by answering these questions:

Are you ready to relieve your painful symptoms and gain back control of your life?

Are you ready to remain symptom free for months, or possibly even years?

Have you been diagnosed with IBS, food sensitives or celiac disease?

Have you been diagnosed with inflammatory irritable bowel disease and have reached a point where your disease is generally well controlled but you still suffer from the appearance of symptoms?

Are you interested in a plan that has been designed to be nutritionally sound and well rounded, specifically created to address the additional needs of people with IBS and other digestive disorders?

Are you looking for a treatment plan that steps outside the box of conventional thinking and approaches healing and alleviation of symptoms from a natural, holistic point of view?

If you have answered "yes" to any of these, I ask you to read further and discover how the four-week, low-FODMAP plan can better your health and change your life.

Chapter 3: Using the Meal Plan, a Rundown of the Basics and Tips for Success

While I believe that knowledge is key, and understanding what FODMAPs are and how they affect your health is an important first step in taking charge of your health, I also know that you are reading this book because you want relief, and you want it as soon as possible. What you want is to get down to the details of the four-week, low-FODMAP plan and learn how you can best introduce it into your life. So, let's get started.

Before you begin your four-week FODMAP adventure, there are a couple of things that I ask you to keep in mind. The first is that it is always best to begin this dietary program, or any other one for that matter, under the counsel of a doctor or nutritionist. This is especially true for people who suffer from IBS, FGID, SIBO and IBDs. Not only are there specific nutritional concerns that might need to be addressed, a qualified professional can also help you identify other factors that should be considered before embarking on a low-FODMAP plan. People who have very inflexible preferences regarding food choices, those who have suffered from or are at risk of eating disorders, those who have dietary restrictions due to other medical conditions and those who already eat a generally low-FODMAP diet should seek additional medical advice to discuss starting, and possibly modifying, this plan to meet your health and nutritional needs.

Recognize that eliminating all potential triggers at once means that you will be temporarily changing not only your dietary habits, but quite possibly your lifestyle as well. One of the downfalls of any diet is the period of adjustment where your body is adjusting to the changes while your mind is still stuck in old patterns of thinking and behavior. Add to it that sometimes there is a period of detoxification where you might notice some new uncomfortable symptoms for a few days. This is especially true if following a low-FODMAP plan drastically changes the types of foods that you typically consume daily.

Starting out on the low-FODMAP plan should not be combined with a change of medications, vitamins or supplements. The reason for this is quite simple. If you are changing or adding a medication, how do you know if the effects on your digestive health are really from the elimination of FODMAPs or from another source? It is best to start the low-FODMAP plan when everything else in your daily routine is stable.

When you decide to commit to a low-FODMAP plan, you really need to go all in, and give 100% of your effort. Since the low-FODMAP plan is an elimination diet, if you introduce just one of the eliminated foods, even just a bite, you need to start over from scratch to achieve the most accurate results.

Think about it for a minute. You have diligently committed to eating only low-FODMAP foods for the past two weeks, and you are starting to notice some changes in how you feel. Then let's say you go out to dinner and in front of you is a basket of fresh from the oven rolls, served with an irresistible honey butter. The smell is intoxicating and your dinner companions are enjoying the treat with abandon. You think to yourself, could one or two bites really hurt? For the sake of the elimination diet, the answer is yes. With just that one bite, you are ingesting multiple FODMAPs. You may or may not have an increase in symptoms from that roll, but if you do, how will you know which of the FODMAPs are to blame. The only solution at this point is to start over by clearing your system of all FODMAPs.

Now that you are mentally prepared to start the low-FODMAP plan, let's get down to the more practical aspects and tips for success.

This low-FODMAP plan includes four weeks' worth of meal plans, shopping lists and delicious recipes for success. You and I both know that any diet is more successful when you are enjoying the foods that you eat. This diet is about more than just losing weight, this diet is about improving your life, and I sincerely want you to succeed. So, I have taken extra care in creating the most delicious, nutritionally balanced low-FODMAP recipes that will appeal to a variety of culinary tastes.

During this initial four-week phase, you will completely eliminate high-FODMAP foods in favor of those on the low-FODMAP list. Your mindset during this phase is paramount. It is important to focus on the delicious alternatives to high-FODMAP foods and how these changes are improving the way you feel, and your outlook on life.

After completing four weeks on the low-FODMAP program, you will begin to reintroduce FODMAPS one at a time. While this phase of the diet is not included in the meal plan, do not worry because this book will supply you with all the tools and advice that you need to navigate through this period. The main thing to remember at this point of the diet is that FODMAPs can only be introduced back into your diet one at a time, so you must be careful to not consume foods that contain multiple FODMAPs unless you have previously reintroduced the other components.

OK, now that we have covered the basics of the plan, let's talk about some tips that will help you to be more successful with this plan.

- Pick a start date. The low-FODMAP plan is not one that most people can just jump into without some planning. If possible, you should start this plan when you have few other obligations that might make sticking to a diet difficult. You should also attempt to start the diet when you are in generally good health, aside from your digestive distress, and do not plan to have a change in medications. Some other considerations for starting the low-FODMAP diet is when you will be able to make an appointment with your doctor, or when you will be able to afford buying special groceries for the duration of four weeks. While many of the foods on the low-FODMAP diet are also low cost, the fact that you might be completely reinventing your daily diet can still be an expense.

- If you live with others, talk to them about the low-FODMAP plan and how they can support you. People who do not suffer from the digestive disorders that the low-FODMAP diet addresses have no need to adjust their diets. Decide beforehand if those close to you are going to make any dietary changes out of solidarity, or if you need to be emotionally prepared to see them enjoying foods that you temporarily can't have.

- If you haven't done so already, a food diary can be your most useful tool on this plan. Food diaries give you a big picture view of how your dietary choices affect the way you feel. You will find this especially important during the reintroduction phase of the plan, so it is a good idea to get into the habit of keeping a food diary now. Your food diary should include everything that you eat, along with what time you ate, how you feel both physically and emotionally, and what time any onset of symptoms occurs. Don't hold back when detailing how you feel on any particular day. Even the smallest details can turn out to be key indicators of your food sensitivities.

- Be prepared for obstacles. There will be times when you will go out to eat, attend a social gathering or just find yourself hungry with a lack of low-FODMAP options. Before you even get started, you should identify your potential trouble areas and address them ahead of time. You can look over the menus at local restaurants and call to ask questions about specific menu items. That way, when dining out becomes a possibility, you are armed with suggestions for restaurants that will cater to your needs. Looking ahead on the calendar will help you identify any special occasions so that you can prepare for them ahead of time. Finally, I have made sure to include a low-FODMAP snack section with recipes for snacks that are shelf stable and can be easily transported and eaten anywhere whenever hunger strikes.

- Go shopping with a list and stick to it. I have provided shopping lists for you in this book that fill the needs of the weekly plans. However, you should decide ahead of time if you are making any modifications to the recipes and adjust the shopping list accordingly. You will be more successful in your shopping ventures, and save money, if you know exactly what you need. If you don't need to wander around browsing shelves for what you think you might need, there is less temptation for cheating, or even making mistakes in your choices.

- Meal prepping can be your friend, especially if you are not used to eating home cooked meals and snacks every day. You can save yourself time and frustration during the week by spending one-day prepping and precooking meals for later in the week.

- Make yourself familiar with the list of high and low-FODMAP foods. In fact, print it out and carry it with you everywhere. Having that resource at your hands is invaluable, and could make or break your success on the plan.

Perhaps the most important tip that I can offer you is to enjoy the experience as much as possible and recognize the low-FODMAP plan for what it is, an opportunity to improve your health and gain freedom from uncomfortable, painful and embarrassing symptoms of IBS and other gastrointestinal disorders. You are doing this for your health, and I promise that you are worth the effort.

Chapter 4: Medical Diagnosis, Creating Your Personalized Plan and Reintroduction

I cannot stress enough that I feel it is very important to consult with a physician before beginning this program, especially if you have not sought medical advice for your digestive issues in the past. Your symptoms might be caused by a food sensitivity to a non-FODMAP food, they might be symptoms of a medical condition that require a higher degree of medical involvement, such as irritable bowel disease, or it could be that your symptoms put together do not indicate that your issues are with FODMAP foods. There could be many possible reasons for your digestive distress, and a doctor can help you determine what exactly is going on and the best treatment plan.

Additionally, the FODMAP plan does eliminate some foods that are generally considered healthy, especially for people who are symptom free. There really is no point in eliminating these foods if you do not need to. A visit with your doctor can help you determine if this really is the best course of action for you. Additionally, you might have special health concerns that would require you to be under medical supervision while following this plan. I can't withhold the information in this book from you until you agree to see a doctor, but I do strongly encourage you to do so before deciding to self-treat with the plan included in this book.

So, what is going to happen once you make an appointment with your doctor? Well, depending on your symptoms, your physician will likely decide to run a few minor tests. A suspicion of more serious conditions, such as IBD, might warrant screening tests such as a colonoscopy; however, if IBS is suspected, your doctor will likely go off a list of diagnostic criteria and perhaps do some simple lab tests.

While the FODMAP diet can help people with a range of digestive disorders, for this section I am going to focus primarily on IBS since this is the condition most commonly eased by the FODMAP plan.

In Chapter 2, we briefly outlined a list of symptoms and diagnostic criteria that your physician would look for before confirming an IBS diagnosis. We also mentioned that IBS is a condition of elimination, which means that other possible reasons for your health issues will need to be eliminated before deciding on an IBS diagnosis. There is a list of "red flag" symptoms that your doctor will look for that could indicate a health condition other than IBS. It is important that if you have any of these symptoms, you should see a doctor rather than self-treating with the FODMAP plan. The red flag symptoms include:

- A family history that include IBD, celiac disease, bowel or ovarian cancer
- Your age at the onset of symptoms. Symptoms of IBS typically onset before the age of 50
- Unexplainable weight loss
- Anemia
- Rectal bleeding
- Masses in the abdominal or rectal area
- Rectal bleeding
- Symptoms severe enough to cause you to wake from sleeping

- Other markers that might indicate inflammatory bowel disease

In some cases, your physician may order the following tests to eliminate other possible causes of your symptoms.

- Full blood count
- Antibody testing
- C-reactive protein
- Red blood cell sedimentation rate
- Plasma viscosity

In some instances, your doctor may order a breath test that can identify the malabsorption of certain FODMAPs including lactose, sorbitol and fructose.

Your FODMAP PLAN

This book is designed to give you guidance on how to best make use of a FODMAP elimination plan. Along with that, you will find a four-week meal plan included. The plan outlined in this book has been designed to be simple and satisfying, so that you do not feel deprived in any way while making your way through the next four weeks.

However, unlike other "diet" books, the aim of this is to help you feel better, not necessarily to help you lose weight, lower your blood pressure or remedy any other health issues than those already mentioned. Because each person is going to have an individual experience with the FODMAP plan, it would be pointless to say that you must follow the plan outlined here exactly. For instance, you might already know that lactose is not one of your triggers, so what would be the point in eliminating it? There really isn't one. The point is for you to eliminate your problem foods. With that in mind, I would like to go through briefly how to modify the plan outline in this book, or how to create a new one for yourself.

First, you should consider how you want to introduce the FODMAP plan into your life. This is probably going to depend a great deal on the severity of your symptoms and your experience with elimination diets in the past. Generally speaking, there are two methods of introducing a low-FODMAP plan into your life. First is through complete elimination and the second is by means of gradual elimination.

The plan outlined in this book is a complete elimination plan. We start you off from day one with not even one of the high-FODMAP foods in your diet. If your symptoms are severe, you are looking for the most complete relief possible, and if you have not done food elimination diets in the past, this is your best place to start.

The complete elimination plan might feel challenging in the beginning, but I assure you that the results you feel will be worth it. Plus, extra care has been put in to creating a meal plan and some accompanying recipes that will make the plan more enjoyable for you.

If you decide to go with the complete, four-week elimination plan, it is very important that you not consume any of the high-FODMAP foods. Even consuming one can throw off your results. This is especially challenging because some of the high-FODMAP foods can be hidden in very unsuspecting places. We will go into this a little more in Chapter 5. While the complete elimination plan is the most challenging, it can also be the most rewarding.

The second way of using the FODMAP elimination plan is by choosing to eliminate one FODMAP group at a time and noticing if you have a reduction in symptoms. This method can be easier; however, you might get incomplete results. For example, you might have a sensitivity to more than one

FODMAP food. If you eliminate only one, you might not experience noticeable relief in your symptoms simply because you are still eating other groups of trigger foods. For this reason, I recommend this style of introduction only to people who already have a good idea of what some of their symptom related triggers are.

When creating this plan, I have tried to keep in mind things like busy lifestyles, the fact that you might be making these meals to share with your family and possibly picky eaters, and other considerations. While this plan is going to work for most people, it might not work for everyone as is, so you might feel like you need to make a few adjustments. This is perfectly fine, if you don't substitute out a low-FODMAP food for one that is higher on the list.

You might want to modify this plan due to culinary preferences, dietary needs and variations in appetites. If you choose to modify, or individualize this plan, or create an entirely new one for yourself, there is a simple set of rules that you should follow to make sure that your individualized plan is nutritionally sound.

- The first rule is to have access to a list of high and low FODMAP foods. One is included in this book; however, you can print one from several sources online or find an app which includes them all and the correct portion size.
- Speaking of portion size, try to keep proper portions in mind. This plan is designed to identify the FODMAP foods that are your sources of distress; however, other factors such as overeating can put additional stress on your digestive system and make it difficult to determine the real source of your symptoms.

- Keep your diet balanced. The FODMAP meal plan can be nutritionally restrictive, so it is important to get as much nutritional value as possible from every meal and snack. Since you will be eliminating most processed foods, it becomes easier to not eat empty calories; however the need to be extra diligent about nutrition is something that you should be aware of.
- You will want to plan for three meals and at least one, if not two, snacks per day. You will want to eat at regular intervals to avoid fluctuations in blood sugar and to ward off cravings.
- It is best to have a meal plan rather than coming up with meal ideas and snacks as you go along.
- It is a good idea to avoid meal planning when you are hungry. If you are hungry, there is a good chance that everything will sound good to you and you might become overzealous in your meal planning adventures. It is best to keep your meal plans simple, with a limited list of ingredients that you are familiar with. An occasional special or culinarily advanced meal is great, but you need to be realistic with yourself about what you will actually be able to do in the kitchen on a daily or weekly basis.
- Repeat the same meals. Everybody has their favorites, right? So, why not repeat them frequently throughout your meal plan? Remember that the low-FODMAP diet is a temporary eating plan. Eventually, you might choose to completely eliminate certain foods, but for now, you are only looking at a period of four weeks before you start the reintroduction phase. Don't be afraid to stick with what is familiar and comfortable, as these will be the meals that will help you to succeed.

Keeping Track of Your Symptoms

Earlier, we made mention of keeping a food diary. I would like to reiterate once again the importance of this step. The point of the FODMAP eating plan is obviously to give you relief from your symptoms, and if you are eliminating all the FODMAP foods, shouldn't you be completely symptom free? Well, perhaps. An overwhelming number of people who do follow this plan for the relief of IBS symptoms do in fact experience significant relief although some symptoms might still be present. You might also be thinking that a food diary is of more importance as you enter the reintroduction phase.

Once you enter the reintroduction phase, it will become extremely important to make note of every possible symptom, regardless of how small. However, keeping a food diary is just as important during the initial elimination phase of the plan as well. Let me tell you why.

First, keeping a food diary now sets you up for good habits in the future. To be honest, keeping a food diary can seem like a tedious task, especially if you go out to eat often. However, the reality is that tracking what you eat and how you feel really takes no more than about five minutes for each meal. This is a small investment considering the possible benefits to your health and how you feel.

If you start your food diary now, you will be more likely to carry the habit with you into the reintroduction phase, which is absolutely vital to fully understanding the impact of FODMAP foods on your health. Also, you might find that there are other non-FODMAP foods that affect your digestive symptoms, or even other aspects of your health. To get the most out of this, you really should approach it from a larger-picture point of view.

Yes, FODMAPs will likely make a tremendous difference in your symptoms, however you should use this opportunity to potentially discover other triggers as well.

When you keep track of the foods you eat in your food diary, you should also be keeping track of your emotional symptoms as well. Are you feeling extra "light" and optimistic today, or is that pounding headache causing some fatigue and irritability? Emotional and mental symptoms are equally important for two reasons. First, some sensitivities to foods can manifest themselves in the form of emotional and mental symptoms, and it is just as important to keep track of these as it is, say abdominal pain and bloating.

Secondly, while the FODMAP plan addresses the effect of certain foods on your digestive health, it has been shown that stress can also be a trigger for symptoms and flare-ups. Keeping track of your emotional wellbeing on a daily basis can possibly help you to notice patterns that contribute to greater levels of stress in your daily life. Reducing this stress can possibly ease your symptoms even more.

Where you keep your food diary is up to you. You might want to keep a small notepad with you all the time, you might choose a gorgeous journal, or you might choose an app or electronic journal to help you with your tracking. Whatever you use, there are certain components that you should always include. These are:

- Time of day.
- Food eaten (including even small amounts, such as a ¼ cup milk added to a main dish meant for several people to share).

- What is going on around you? Is this a quick bite by yourself in the kitchen, a celebration, or a lunch with coworkers?
- How you are feeling. Note any symptoms that you might have before eating, including physical, mental and emotional symptoms. Rate them on a scale of 1-10.
- How do you feel afterward? Note any symptoms that you notice and rate them on a scale of 1-10. Realize that not all symptoms occur at the same time, so you might need to come back and add them in. You should also make note of the duration of time that passed between when you ate and the onset of symptoms.
- Review your food diary once a week. On a separate page of your food diary, make note of any patterns that you notice.
- While this FODMAP plan is designed to start with a complete elimination of FODMAP foods before the reintroduction phase, you may choose to do a partial elimination before starting. Your food diary can help you identify trigger foods to eliminate.

The Reintroduction Phase

After four weeks of eliminating high-FODMAP foods, you will begin a period of reintroduction. This allows you to reintroduce each FODMAP food individually while your diet otherwise consists of low-FODMAP foods. The intended result is that you have eliminated these foods from your diet for a long enough period of time that the reintroduction of each food should cause some noticeable symptoms if it is a trigger food for you.

Of course, after a period of elimination when you are feeling great, you are bound to ask yourself "why reintroduce these foods when I feel so great without them in my life?" There is a two-part answer to this question.

The first is if you don't gradually begin to reintroduce these foods back into your diet, you will never know for sure which ones might be triggers for you. Secondly, your gut might actually need small doses of high-FODMAP foods. Let me tell you why.

Within your gut is a population of microbes, or bacteria, that is important not only for digestive function but for your overall health. The very same fermentation that can cause your unpleasant symptoms is the same fermentation that normally feeds the good bacteria in your gut. Without a proper food source, some of the good bacteria can die off, resulting in an imbalance. Many of the foods on the high-FODMAP list can be considered probiotics, which means that they either introduce healthy bacteria into the gut, or provide the food to sustain it. Following the low-FODMAP plan for just four weeks can be enough to disrupt the balance, which can eventually cause worse symptoms.

The remedy to this is to supply small amounts of these foods in order to maintain that proper balance. As you reintroduce the eliminated foods, you slowly help to rebalance your system. Most people find that once they have eliminated a trigger food, they can occasionally eat small amounts without digestive disturbance. The theory behind this is that your body reaches a threshold of how much it can handle before a flare-up of symptoms develops. Following this theory, it is possible that you will be able to occasionally enjoy small amounts of high-FODMAP foods, as long as you do not overindulge or include them in your diet regularly. Additionally, once you know which FODMAP foods aren't a cause of your symptoms, you can safely include them in your diet to help support proper gut health.

After completing the four-week plan, use the following steps as a guideline to reintroduce the FODMAP foods into your diet.

- Choose a FODMAP group to begin with. The oligosaccharides are a good group to begin with because they are high in prebiotic fibers, which will help to rebuild your gut bacteria the fastest.
- Secondly, choose a specific food from the chosen group to reintroduce. The Monash University, where the FODMAP diet was first researched, has an app available that will help you determine the correct portion of high-FODMAP foods to consume for reintroduction.
- Remember, only one high-FODMAP group at a time. It is especially important to maintain an otherwise low-FODMAP diet while reintroducing foods.
- Give it some time. You might experience symptoms almost immediately; however, it might take up to 48 hours before any symptoms present themselves. Make sure to keep track of how you feel using your food diary during this period.
- If, after 48 hours, you do not experience any negative symptoms, you can try again with the same food, except with a larger portion. Again, give it about 48 hours to see if any symptoms develop.
- After your first reintroduction, give yourself a 24-hour period of low-FODMAP eating before you try reintroducing another FODMAP group.

Now, that we have covered what FODMAPs are, what a low-FODMAP eating plan is and how it can affect your health, and if you are a good candidate for this eating plan, it is time to actually get started. In the next chapter, we will go through a comprehensive list of high and low FODMAP foods, along with the suggested for week FODMAP elimination plan.

Chapter 5: The Low-FODMAP Meal Plan in Action

The number one tool that you will need for the next four weeks, aside from a little willpower and a desire to feel better, is a comprehensive list of low and high-FODMAP foods. We tend to think that only "junk" foods are bad for us and our digestive health, but for people with IBS and other digestive disorders, the truth is that sometimes very healthy foods are some of the worst culprits.

Therefore, it is important to not make any assumptions about which foods are safe to eat during this elimination plan. Get familiar with this list because it is going to be your guideline for symptom relief during the next four weeks.

High FODMAP FOODS for Elimination
Vegetables

- Asparagus
- Artichokes
- Beet root
- Cassava
- Cauliflower
- Celery
- Garlic, including garlic salt
- Leek
- Legumes/ pulses (baked beans, black beans, black eyed peas, broad beans, butter beans, kidney beans, haricot beans, lima beans, mung beans, soy beans, split peas)

- Mushrooms
- Onions (red, yellow, white, spring and green onions)
- Onion powder and salt
- Pickled vegetables
- Sauerkraut
- Savoy cabbage
- Scallions
- Shallots
- Sugar snap peas
- Sweet corn
- Taro

Fruits

- Apples
- Apricots
- Avocado
- Blackberries
- Blackcurrants
- Boysenberry
- Cherries
- Currants
- Dates
- Figs
- Goji berries
- Grapefruit
- Guava
- Lychee
- Nectarines
- Nashi pears
- Peaches
- Pears
- Plums

- Watermelon

Dairy

- Buttermilk
- Cow's milk
- Cream
- Custard
- Evaporated milk
- Goats milk
- Ice cream
- Kefir
- Soft cheeses (cream cheese, ricotta cheese, etc.)

**The key to knowing if a cheese is a low FODMAP food is in looking at the label. First, check to make sure there are no added sugars on the ingredient label. Once you verify that no sugar has been added, check the nutritional label for the amount of sugars per serving. Lactose, will show up as a sugar in cheese products. If the cheese has 1g of sugar or less per serving, it is considered a low FODMAP food. Cheeses with slightly more than this are a moderately low FODMAP food and should be used only in moderation. Avoid cheeses that contain more than 2g of sugar per serving. The above list is only a representation of possible low to moderately low FODMAP cheese choices. The actual level can vary from one producer to the next, so check the sugar levels to make sure, even for the cheeses included on this list.

- Sour cream
- Yogurt

Protein

- Legumes/pulses (baked beans, black beans, black eyed peas, broad beans, butter beans, kidney beans, haricot beans, lima beans, mung beans, soy beans, split peas)
- Chorizo
- Sausage

Grains

- Wheat, including wheat containing breads, cereal, pasta, crackers and other baked goods.
- Rye, including rye containing breads, cereal, pasta, crackers and other baked goods.
- Amaranth
- Barley
- Bran
- Couscous
- Semolina
- spelt

Nuts and Seeds

- Cashews
- Pistachios

Condiments, Sweeteners, Etc.

- Agave
- Fructose
- Fruit bar
- Prepared gravy containing onion
- High fructose corn syrup (HFCS)
- Hummus

- Honey
- Jam
- Pesto
- Relish
- Stock cubes
- Sugar free foods that contain polyols – usually ending in -ol or isomalt
- Sweeteners:
- Inulin
- Isomalt
- Maltitol
- Mannitol
- Sorbitol
- Xylitol
- Tahini paste

Beverages

- Alcohol (wine, beer and spirits)
- Fruit juice of any of the fruits listed above
- Teas that contain any of the fruits listed above
- Soy drinks
- Sports drinks
- Sodas
- Lactose containing whey protein

Low FODMAP Foods for Inclusion

*Denotes foods that are acceptable in limited amounts. Maximum daily quantities are listed.

Vegetables

- Alfalfa
- Baby spinach
- Bamboo shoots
- Bean sprouts
- Bok choy
- Broccoli* (½ cup)
- Brussel sprouts* (¼ cup)
- Butter lettuce
- Butternut squash* (¼ cup)
- Cabbage, green and red * (1 cup)
- Carrots
- Chick peas* (¼ cup)
- Chives
- Collard greens
- Cucumber
- Eggplant
- Fennel
- Green beans
- Green pepper
- Ginger
- Iceberg lettuce
- Kale
- Lentils* (¼ cup)
- Okra
- Parsnip
- Potato
- Pumpkin
- Radicchio

- Radish
- Red peppers
- Seaweed
- Snow peas* (¼ cup)
- Spaghetti squash
- Squash
- Swiss chard
- Sweet potato* (½ cup)
- Tomato
- Turnip
- Water chestnuts
- Yam
- Zucchini

Fruits

- Bananas
- Blueberries
- Breadfruit
- Cantaloupe
- Clementine
- Dragon fruit
- Lingonberries
- Grapes
- Guava
- Honeydew
- Kiwi
- Lemon
- Lime
- Mandarin oranges
- Orange
- Passion fruit
- Papaya

- Pineapple
- Plantain
- Raspberry
- Rhubarb
- Strawberry
- Tamarind

Dairy

- Almond milk
- Butter
- Cheeses including brie, camembert, cheddar, cottage cheese, feta cheese, goat, mozzarella, parmesan, swiss.
  **The key to knowing if a cheese is a low FODMAP food is in looking at the label. First, check to make sure there are no added sugars on the ingredient label. Once you verify that no sugar has been added, check the nutritional label for the amount of sugars per serving. Lactose, will show up as a sugar in cheese products. If the cheese has 1g of sugar or less per serving, it is considered a low FODMAP food. Cheeses with slightly more than this are a moderately low FODMAP food and should be used only in moderation. Avoid cheeses that contain more than 2g of sugar per serving. The above list is only a representation of possible low to moderately low FODMAP cheese choices. The actual level can vary from one producer to the next, so check the sugar levels to make sure, even for the cheeses included on this list.
- Eggs
- Hemp milk
- Lactose free milk

- Margarine
- Rice milk* (½ cup)
- Tempeh
- Lactose free yogurt

Protein

- Beef
- Chicken
- Lamb
- Pork
- Turkey
- Cold cuts (ham, chicken, turkey, etc.)
- Canned tuna
- Cod
- Salmon
- Trout
- Tuna
- Crab
- Lobster
- Mussels
- Oysters
- Prawns
- Shrimp

Grains

- Corn bread
- Potato flour bread
- Wheat free oat bread
- Wheat free pasta
- Wheat free or gluten free pasta
- Bulgur* (½ cup)

- Buckwheat
- Brown rice
- Corn tortillas
- Millet
- Oatmeal (½ cup)
- Oats
- Polenta
- Quinoa
- Basmati rice
- White rice
- Rice cakes
- Rice flour
- Sorghum

Nuts and Seeds

- Almonds
- Brazil nuts
- Chestnuts
- Hazelnuts
- Macadamia nuts
- Peanuts
- Pecans
- Pine nuts
- Walnuts
- Chia seeds
- Poppy seeds
- Pumpkin seeds
- Sesame seeds
- Sunflower seeds

Condiments, Sweeteners, Etc.

- Aspartame
- Capers
- Dark chocolate
- Chocolate:
- Glucose
- Ketchup
- Maple syrup
- Marmalade
- Mayonnaise
- Miso paste
- Mustard
- Oyster sauce
- Peanut butter
- Rice malt syrup
- Saccharine
- Soy sauce
- Stevia
- Sucralose
- Sugar
- Tamarind paste
- Apple cider vinegar* (1/8 cup)
- Balsamic vinegar* (1/8 cup)
- Rice wine vinegar
- Wasabi
- Oils: avocado oil, canola oil, coconut oil, olive oil, peanut oil, sesame oil, sunflower oil, vegetable oil

Beverages

- Coffee
- White tea, black tea, green tea, peppermint tea

- Carbonated water
- Fruit juice from low FODMAP fruits
- Aspartame sweetened beverages (small amounts)
- Water

Weekly Meal Plans

Snack and desserts are encouraged on the low-FODMAP plan. However, they have not been included in these daily meal plans because they are optional. You can find some great ideas and recipes for snacks and desserts in the recipes section of this book.

Denotes meals suggestions with recipes included in this book.

Week 1

The first week on the low-FODMAP plan should be about simplicity and familiarity. Remember that being overly ambitious at the beginning of any diet plan and become a setup for burnout. Take it easy this week and ease your way into the low-FODMAP plan by choosing foods from the approved list that are your favorites and normal staples.

Day 1:

- Breakfast: Breakfast Burritos
- **Lunch: Creamy Stuffed Potatoes*** with garden salad
- Dinner: Roast Beef and vegetables

Day 2:

- Breakfast: Scrambled eggs with chilled cooked salmon
- **Lunch: Chef Salad*** and fresh berries
- Dinner: Grilled Chicken over steamed greens and rice

Day 3:

- Breakfast: Banana Blueberry Smoothie and ½ cup cooked oats
- **Lunch: Asian Chicken and Rice Bowl***
- **Dinner: Scented pork stir fry***

Day 4:

- **Breakfast: Maple Spice Chia Breakfast Pudding*** and fresh strawberries
- Lunch: Grilled Tomato and Cheese on Gluten Free Wheat Free Bread, and garden salad
- **Dinner: Chicken Fajita Plate***

Day 5:

- Breakfast: Breakfast Burritos
- Lunch: Tuna Salad in Iceberg Lettuce Cups with fresh pineapple
- **Dinner: Sesame Beef and rice***

Day 6:

- Breakfast: Poach eggs over Sautéed Collard Greens
- **Lunch: Brie Caprese Style Polenta***
- **Dinner: Lemon Butter Shrimp over Vegetable Noodles***

Day 7:

- **Breakfast: Banana Split French Toast***
- **Lunch: Fajita Salad***

- **Dinner: Stuffed Peppers*** and sautéed spinach with walnuts

Week 2

Day 1:

- Breakfast: Baby Spinach and Brie Omelet
- Lunch: Ham, Swiss and Tomato on Gluten Free Bread and garden salad
- **Dinner: Cajun Steak and Twice Baked Potatoes*** with steamed green beans

Day 2:

- Breakfast: Breakfast Burritos
- **Lunch: Creamy Stuffed Potatoes*** and garden salad
- **Dinner: Lemon Ginger Chicken and Rice Soup***

Day 3:

- Breakfast: Oats with cinnamon and Orange and 1-piece FODMAP approved gluten free toast with small amount of butter
- **Lunch: Quinoa Salad*** and low- FODMAP fruit selection
- Dinner: Baked Chicken with Braised Radicchio

Day 4:

- **Breakfast: Blueberry Lemon Scones*** and almond milk latte
- **Lunch: Pineapple Chicken Skewers*** and cooked quinoa
- Dinner: Salmon, Vegetables and Rice

Day 5:

- Breakfast: Eggs with lean turkey
- **Lunch: Italian Rice Bowl***
- **Dinner: Curry Chicken Stew***

Day 6:

- **Breakfast: Orange Essence French Toast***
- **Lunch: Chef Salad***
- Dinner: Stuffed Pork Loin, roasted carrots and sautéed brussels sprouts with walnuts

Day 7:

- Breakfast: Fruit Salad and Brie
- **Lunch: Gingered Carrot Soup***
- Dinner: One Pot Chicken Tacos

Week 3

Day 1:

- Breakfast: Breakfast Burritos
- Lunch: Fruit and Brie plate
- **Dinner: Simple Beef Stew***

Day 2:

- Breakfast: Veggie and Cheddar Omelet
- **Lunch: Rustic Potato Soup***
- **Dinner: Pineapple Shrimp Fajitas***

Day 3:

- **Breakfast: Tropical Smoothie *** and ¼ cup almonds
- Lunch: Chicken Stir fry
- Dinner: Stuffed Peppers and Green Salad

Day 4:

- **Breakfast: Vanilla Walnut Oatmeal*** and 1 egg cooked to liking
- **Lunch: Fruited Chicken Salad***
- Dinner: Green vegetable and rice skillet

Day 5:

- Breakfast: Blueberry, Walnut and Cheese plate
- **Lunch: Fajita Salad***
- **Dinner: Simple Beef Stew***

Day 6:

- Breakfast: Egg, Tomato and Baby Spinach Stack
- Lunch: Green Power Smoothie and Mixed Nuts
- Dinner: Not Quite Thanksgiving Dinner (roasted turkey, polenta, green beans and raspberry sauce)

Day 7:

- Breakfast: Breakfast Burritos
- Lunch: Caprese Salad (baby spinach, tomatoes, compliant mozzarella or brie, fresh basil, vinegar)
- Dinner: Chicken with **Fruit Sauce*** with braised collard greens

Week 4

Day 1:

- Breakfast: Raspberry Vanilla Smoothie and 1 egg on FODMAP approved gluten free toast
- Lunch: Triple Cheese Grilled Sandwich on Gluten Free Bread and garden salad
- **Dinner: Lemon Butter Shrimp over Vegetable Noodles***

Day 2:

- **Breakfast: Papaya Chia Breakfast Pudding*** and fresh blueberries and strawberries
- **Lunch: Asian Rice Bowl***
- **Dinner: Maple Salmon*** with quinoa and roasted carrots

Day 3:

- Breakfast: Vegetable Omelet
- Lunch: Grilled Chicken and Vegetables
- Dinner: Extreme Veggie and Cheese Sandwiches on Gluten Free Bread, garden salad

Day 4:

- Breakfast: Breakfast Burritos
- **Lunch: Fruit and Protein Salad***
- **Dinner: Simple Beef Stew***

Day 5:

- Breakfast: **Blueberry Lemon Scones*** and 1 egg cooked to liking
- **Lunch: Creamy Stuffed Potatoes*** with simple chicken broth
- Dinner: Meatloaf with Grilled Bok Choy

Day 6:

- **Breakfast: Banana Split French Toast**
- **Lunch: Quinoa Salad***
- Dinner: Ginger Chicken Stir Fry

Day 7:

- Breakfast: Fruit Salad with Brie
- Lunch: **Salmon Patties with Caper Mayonnaise*** with Fresh Salad
- **Dinner: Swiss Stuffed Chicken*** and grilled bok choy

Chapter 6: **Low-FODMAP Recipes for Every Meal and Every Occasion**

Breakfasts

Maple Spice Chia Breakfast Pudding

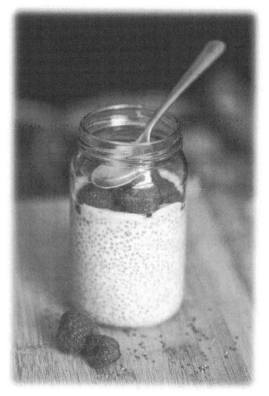

Servings: 4

Ingredients:
- 2 cups almond milk
- ½ cup chia seeds
- 3 tablespoons pure maple syrup

- ½ teaspoon ground cinnamon
- ¼ teaspoon ground nutmeg
- 1 teaspoon orange zest
- ¼ cup almonds, chopped or sliced
- Raspberries for garnish, optional

Directions:

1. In a bowl, combine the almond milk, pure maple syrup, cinnamon, nutmeg and orange zest. Mix well.
2. Stir in the chia seeds.
3. Cover and place in the refrigerator for at least 4 hours or overnight.
4. Serve topped with chopped or sliced almonds, and raspberries, if desired.

Banana Split French Toast

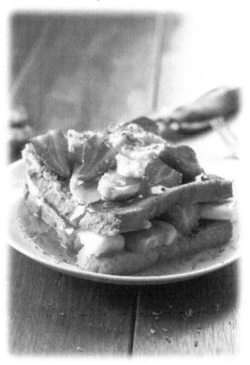

Servings: 4

Ingredients:

- 8 slices gluten free bread, or other low fodmap bread choice
- 3 eggs
- 1 teaspoon ground cinnamon
- ½ teaspoon ground ginger
- 2 tablespoons butter
- 1 medium banana, sliced
- 1 cup fresh strawberries, sliced
- ½ cup fresh pineapples, chopped
- ½ cup walnuts, chopped
- Pure maple syrup (optional)

Directions:

1. Whisk the eggs, cinnamon and ginger in a bowl until creamy.
2. Place the 1 tablespoon of the butter in a skillet over medium heat.
3. Once the skillet is hot, take one piece of bread and dip it in the egg mixture. Remove, turn over and dip again, so that both sides of the bread are coated.
4. Place the bread in the skillet and cook for approximately 3 minutes per side, or until browned.
5. Repeat with the remaining pieces of bread, add the additional butter when necessary to oil the skillet.
6. Place one slice of French toast on each serving plate. Top that piece with the sliced bananas and then a second piece of the French toast.
7. Top with fresh strawberries, pineapple and pure maple syrup, if desired.

Blueberry Lemon Scones

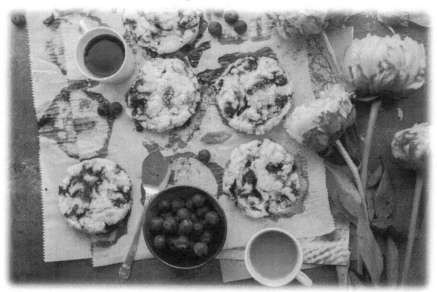

Servings: 6 (2 scones per serving)

Ingredients:

- 1 cup rice flour
- ½ cup cornmeal
- 1 tablespoon baking powder
- 1 tablespoon brown sugar
- 1 teaspoon ground ginger
- ¼ cup butter, chilled and cubed
- ¼ cup almond milk or appropriate lactose free alternative
- 1 egg
- 1 cup fresh blueberries
- 2 tablespoons lemon juice
- 2 teaspoons lemon zest

Directions:

1. Preheat the oven to 400°F.
2. In one bowl, mix together the rice flour, cornmeal, baking powder, brown sugar, and ground ginger.
3. In a separate bowl, whisk together the almond milk, egg, lemon juice and lemon zest.
4. Take the chilled butter and work it into the flour mixture with your hands until the mixture is crumbly.
5. Add the almond milk and egg mixture to the flour mixture and mix just until blended.
6. Fold in the blueberries.
7. Transfer the dough out onto a lightly floured countertop. The dough will be crumbly.
8. Gently press the dough together while pressing it down, forming a rectangle that is about 1 inch thick.
9. Cut the dough into 12 equally sized squares and then transfer them onto a baking sheet.
10. Place in the oven for 15-20 minutes, or until risen and golden brown.
11. Remove from the oven and allow to cool before serving. Store uneaten scones in an airtight container.

Orange Essence French Toast

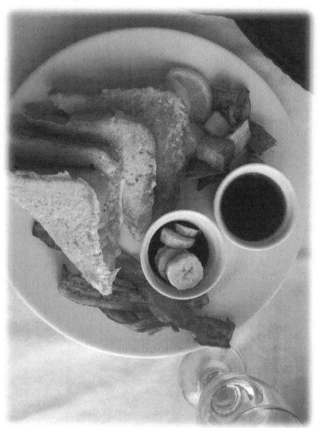

Servings: 4

Ingredients:
- 8 slices gluten free, FODMAP approved bread
- 3 eggs
- ½ cup orange juice
- 2 teaspoons orange zest
- ½ teaspoon pure vanilla extract
- ½ teaspoon cinnamon
- Pure maple syrup (optional)

Directions:

1. In a bowl, combine the eggs, orange juice, orange zest, pure vanilla extract and cinnamon. Whisk until blended and creamy.
2. Heat one tablespoon of the butter in a skillet over medium heat.
3. Once the butter in the skillet is hot, take each piece of bread and dip it into the egg mixture. Turn the bread over and dip in the egg mixture again, to make sure that both sides are equally coated.
4. Place the pieces of bread in the skillet and cook for approximately 3 minutes per side, or until browned. Add more butter to the skillet as necessary to keep it greased.
5. Remove the French toast from the skillet and serve with pure maple syrup, if desired.

Tropical Smoothie

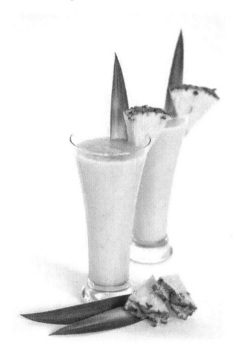

Servings: 2

Ingredients:
- 1 frozen banana, sliced
- 1 cup fresh pineapple
- 1 cup fresh or frozen papaya chunks
- 1 cup orange juice
- Ice

Directions:

1. Combine all the ingredients in a blender, and blend until smooth.
2. Transfer to well chilled glasses for serving.

Vanilla Walnut Oatmeal

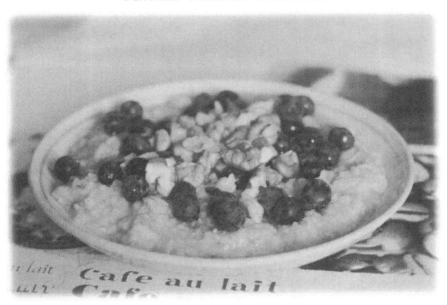

Servings: 4

Ingredients:

- 1 cup quick cooking oats
- 3-4 cups water (depending on package directions)
- 1 tablespoon chia seeds
- 1 vanilla bean, scraped
- 1 ½ teaspoons cinnamon
- ½ cup almond milk
- ½ cup walnuts, chopped

Directions:

1. In a microwave safe bowl, combine the quick cooking oats, water, vanilla and cinnamon.
2. Cook in the microwave for approximately 5 minutes, or until the water is absorbed and the oats are tender. Check package instructions on your individual brand.

3. Remove the oatmeal from the microwave, stir in the chia seeds and transfer to individual serving dishes.
4. Top with almond milk and walnuts before serving.

Papaya Chia Breakfast Pudding

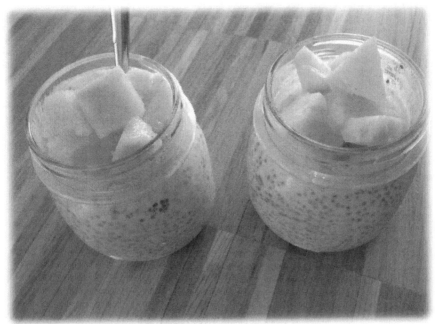

Servings: 4

Ingredients:

- 2 cups almond milk
- ½ cup chia seeds
- ½ cup papaya, pureed
- 1 tablespoon orange juice

Directions:

1. In a bowl, combine the almond milk, papaya and orange juice. Mix well.
2. Stir in the chia seeds.
3. Cover and refrigerate for at least 4 hours, or overnight before serving.

Lunch

Creamy Stuffed Potatoes

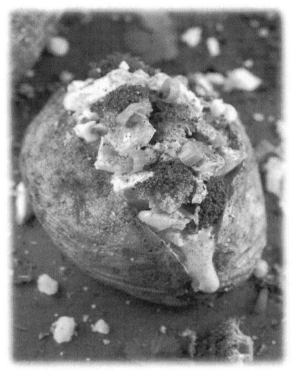

Servings: 4

Ingredients:

- 4 medium sized baking potatoes
- 1 cup cottage cheese (check label for sugar content. See note about cheeses on the low-FODMAP food list)
- 1 cup broccoli, chopped
- 1 cup cooked chicken, shredded
- ¼ cup sunflower seeds
- 1 teaspoon olive oil

Directions:

1. Wash the baking potatoes and pierce little holes over the surface using a fork.
2. Place the potatoes in a microwave safe dish and cook in the microwave for 7-10 minutes, depending on the size of the potatoes and the wattage, until the potatoes are tender.
3. Meanwhile, heat the oil in a skillet over medium heat.
4. Add the broccoli and season with a pinch of salt and pepper, if desired.
5. Cook the broccoli until tender.
6. Add the chicken to the skillet and cook just until warmed through.
7. Remove the potatoes from the microwave and carefully transfer them to serving plates.
8. Slice open each potato and carefully pull it open.
9. Place a portion of the cottage cheese into each potato, followed by the chicken and broccoli.
10. Top with sunflower seeds before serving.

Asian Chicken and Rice Bowl

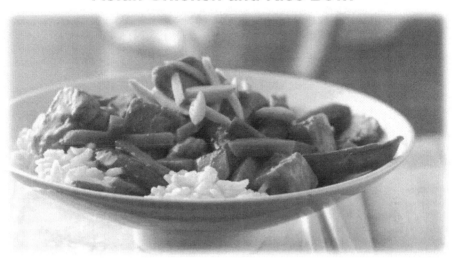

Servings: 4

Ingredients:

- 1 lb. boneless skinless chicken breast, sliced thin
- 1 ½ cups red bell pepper, sliced
- 6 cups fresh spinach, chopped
- ½ cup water chestnuts
- 1 tablespoon sesame oil
- ¼ cup soy sauce
- 1 tablespoon fresh grated ginger
- ½ teaspoon black pepper
- ½ cup peanuts, chopped
- 1 tablespoon sesame seeds
- 3 cups hot cooked basmati rice

Directions:

1. Heat the sesame oil in a skillet over medium to medium high heat.

2. Add the chicken and season it with the black pepper. Cook for 2 minutes.
3. Next, add in the red bell pepper and continue cooking for 2-3 minutes.
4. Add in the spinach, water chestnuts, and fresh grated ginger.
5. Sprinkle in the soy sauce and continue cooking until the spinach is wilted and the chicken is cooked through.
6. Serve the chicken and vegetable mixture over hot cooked basmati rice.
7. Garnish with sesame seeds and chopped peanuts before serving.

Brie Caprese Style Polenta

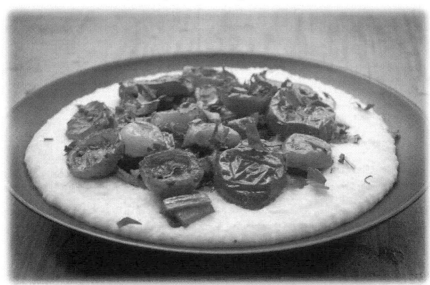

Servings: 4

Ingredients:

- 1 cup polenta
- 3 cups water or chicken broth
- ½ cup brie, cubed
- 1 tablespoon butter
- ½ teaspoon salt
- ½ teaspoon black pepper
- 1 tablespoon olive oil
- 1 medium tomato, sliced
- ½ cup fresh basil, chopped

Directions:

1. Preheat the oven to 350°F and line a baking sheet with aluminum foil.

2. Place the water or chicken broth in a large saucepan over medium heat.
3. Once the water warms, reduce the heat to medium low and stir in the polenta.
4. Continue cooking, stirring frequently to prevent sticking, for approximately 20 minutes, or until the polenta thickens.
5. While the polenta is cooking, place the tomato slices on the baking sheet and drizzle them with olive oil.
6. Place the baking sheet in the oven and bake for 10 minutes. Remove and set aside.
7. Season the polenta with the salt and black pepper. Add the butter and the brie and stir until the brie begins to melt into the polenta.
8. Transfer the polenta to serving dishes and top with the roasted tomato slices and fresh basil.

Italian Rice Bowl

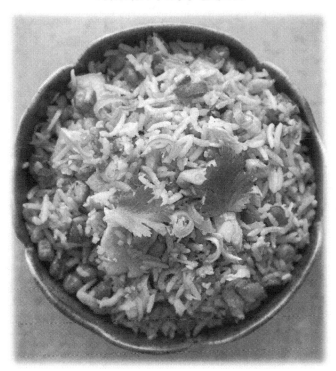

Servings: 4

Ingredients:

- 1 tablespoon olive oil
- 1 cup long grain white rice
- 2 cups chicken broth (homemade or low-FODMAP)
- ½ teaspoon salt
- ½ teaspoon black pepper
- ¼ cup fresh basil, chopped
- ¼ fresh grated parmesan
- ½ lb. cooked, shredded chicken
- 2 cups radicchio, shredded or cut into strips
- 1 cup roasted red bell peppers

Directions:

1. Heat the olive oil in a skillet over medium heat.
2. Add the rice and cook while stirring until the rice is lightly toasted.
3. Add in the chicken broth, salt, and black pepper.
4. Increase the heat to medium high and bring the liquid to a boil.
5. Reduce the heat to low, cover and simmer for 20 minutes, or until the liquid is absorbed
6. Meanwhile, add a little more olive oil in a separate skillet.
7. Add in the radicchio and sauté for 5-7 minutes, or until it becomes tender. Add in the roasted red peppers and the chicken. Continue cooking, until warmed through.
8. Remove the lid from the rice and stir in the basil and the parmesan.
9. Transfer the rice to serving bowls and top with the chicken and vegetable mixture.

Pineapple Chicken Skewers

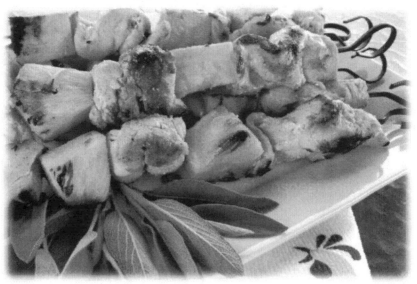

Servings: 4

Ingredients:

- 1 lb. boneless skinless chicken tenders, cut into cubes
- ¼ cup soy sauce
- 1 tablespoon brown sugar
- 2 teaspoons lime juice
- 2 teaspoons fresh grated ginger
- 1 cup fresh pineapple chunks
- 1 cup green bell pepper, cut into chunks
- 1 cup tomato, cut into chunks
- Metal or bamboo skewers

Directions:

1. Begin by combining the soy sauce, brown sugar, lime juice and ginger in a bowl.
2. Add the chicken and let marinate for 30 minutes or longer in the refrigerator.

3. Meanwhile, if you are using bamboo skewers, soak them in water for at least 15 minutes before using to prevent burning.
4. Preheat and indoor or outdoor grill over medium heat.
5. Using an alternating pattern, place pieces of the chicken, pineapple, bell pepper and tomato on each skewer, making sure to leave a little bit of room between each addition to ensure even cooking.
6. Place the skewers on the grill and cook for 5-6 minutes per side, depending on the size of the chicken pieces, or until the chicken is cooked through.

Salads

Fajita Salad

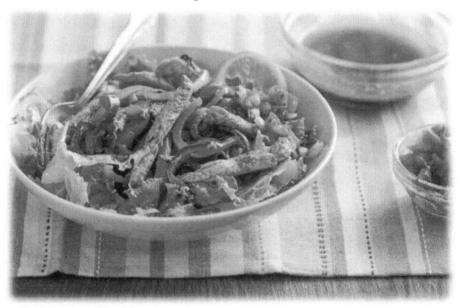

Servings: 4

Ingredients:

- 1 tablespoon olive oil
- 2 cups red bell peppers, sliced
- 2 cups zucchini, sliced
- ½ teaspoon salt
- ½ teaspoon black pepper
- 1 cup tomatoes, diced
- 6 cups baby spinach
- ¾ lb. cooked chicken, shredded and warmed
- 1 cup crushed tortilla chips (check ingredients for FODMAP approval)
- Southwest Fajita Dressing (see recipe)

Directions:

1. Heat the olive oil in a skillet over medium heat.
2. Once the oil is hot, add in the red bell peppers and zucchini. Cooke the vegetables for approximately 5 minutes, or until the vegetables are firm tender.
3. Add the baby spinach to the serving plates and drizzle with the Southwest Fajita Dressing.
4. Next, sprinkle on the crushed tortilla chips, followed by the sautéed vegetables and chicken.

Quinoa Salad

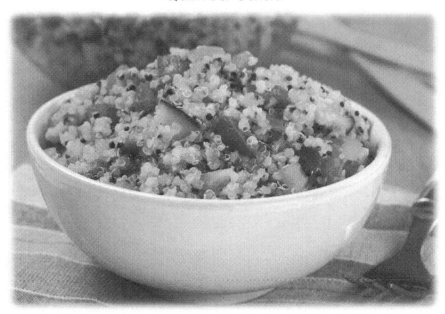

Servings: 4

Ingredients:
- 1 cup quinoa
- 2 cups water or FODMAP approved broth
- 3 tablespoons olive oil
- 1 ½ tablespoons lemon juice
- ¼ cup pine nuts
- ¾ cup roasted red peppers, chopped
- 1 cup kale, finely chopped
- ¾ cup feta cheese, crumbled
- ¼ cup fresh basil, chopped
- ½ teaspoon salt
- ½ teaspoon black pepper

Directions:

1. Combine the quinoa and water or broth in a saucepan over medium high heat.
2. Once the liquid comes to a boil, reduce the heat to low, cover and simmer for 15-20 minutes.
3. Remove the cover from the saucepan, fluff the quinoa and transfer it to a large bowl.
4. Whisk together the olive oil, lemon juice, salt and black pepper.
5. Drizzle the dressing over the quinoa and stir.
6. Add in the pine nuts, roasted red peppers, feta cheese and basil. Mix well.
7. Serve warm or cover and refrigerate until ready to serve.

Fruited Chicken Salad

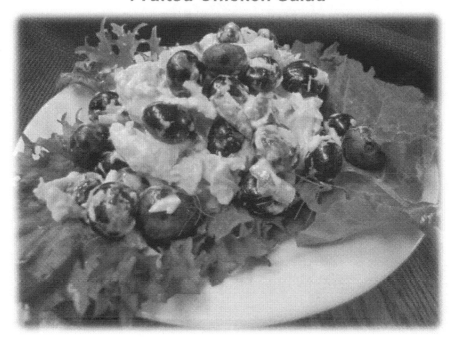

Servings: 4

Ingredients:

- 6 cups baby spinach leaves
- ½ cup raspberries, halved
- ¾ cup blueberries
- 1 cup mandarin orange slices
- 3 tablespoons mayonnaise (check ingredients for FODMAP compliance)
- 2 tablespoons olive oil
- 1 teaspoon stone ground mustard
- ¼ cup feta cheese
- 2 tablespoons fresh mint
- ½ lb. cooked chicken, shredded or cubed
- ½ cup walnuts, chopped

Directions:

1. In a blender or food processor, combine the mayonnaise, olive oil, stone ground mustard, feta cheese, and mint. Blend until creamy.
2. In a bowl, spinach, raspberries, blueberries and mandarin orange slices. Toss to mix.
3. Place the salad mixture on individual serving plates.
4. In a separate bowl, combine the chicken and the dressing. Mix well.
5. Place equal sized portions of the dressed chicken on the salad.
6. Top with walnuts before serving.

Chef Salad

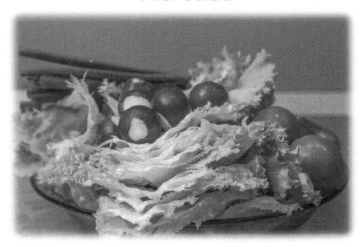

Servings: 4

Ingredients:

- 6 cups butter lettuce, torn
- 1 ½ cups cooked turkey, cubed
- 2 eggs, hardboiled and halved
- ½ cup canned chickpeas, rinsed and drained
- ½ cup cucumber, sliced
- ½ cup radishes, sliced thin
- ¾ cup tomatoes, diced
- ¼ cup pumpkin seeds
- Caper Dressing (see recipe)

Directions:

1. Divide the butter lettuce among the serving dishes.
2. Dress the salad greens with the caper dressing.
3. Arrange the turkey, chickpeas, cucumber, radishes and tomatoes on top of the salad in rows.
4. Garnish the salad with one half of a hardboiled egg and pumpkin seeds before serving.

Fruit and Protein Salad

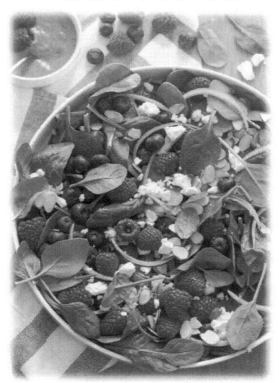

Servings: 4

Ingredients:

- 6 cups baby spinach
- 2 cup cooked turkey, cubed or sliced
- ½ cup brussels sprouts, shaved
- 1 tablespoon olive oil
- ½ teaspoon salt
- ½ teaspoon black pepper
- 1 cup blueberries
- ½ cup feta cheese
- ½ cup walnuts
- Raspberry Citrus Vinaigrette (see recipe)

Directions:

1. Heat the olive oil in a skillet over medium heat.
2. Once the oil is hot, add the brussels sprouts and season them with the salt and black pepper.
3. Sauté the shredded brussels sprouts for approximately 4-5 minutes, or until tender.
4. Remove the skillet from the heat and set aside.
5. In a bowl, combine the spinach, turkey, blueberries, and feta cheese.
6. Drizzle the salad Raspberry Citrus Vinaigrette over the salad and toss.
7. Transfer the salad to individual serving plates.
8. Top with the sautéed brussels sprouts and walnuts before serving.

Gingered Carrot Soup

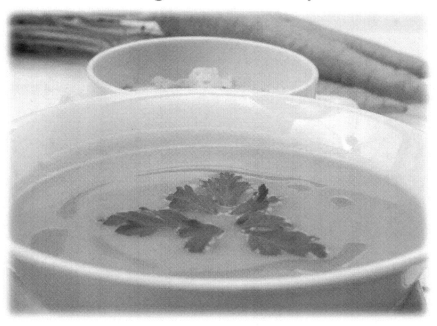

Servings: 4-6

Ingredients:

- 2 tablespoons butter
- 1 lb. carrots, peeled and diced
- 2 tablespoons fresh grated ginger
- ½ teaspoon salt
- ½ teaspoon black pepper
- ½ teaspoon cinnamon
- ½ teaspoon nutmeg
- 4 cups chicken or vegetable broth (FODMAP compliant)
- 1 cup cooked pumpkin, mashed

- 1 cup almond milk, or other FODMAP compliant milk alternative
- ¼ cup walnuts, chopped
- ¼ cup fresh parsley, chopped

Directions:

1. Add the butter to a large soup pan or stockpot.
2. Once the butter is hot, add in the carrots, salt, black pepper, cinnamon and nutmeg and sauté, stirring occasionally for 5-7 minutes or until tender.
3. Add the ginger and cook 1-2 additional minutes
4. Add in the broth, and increase the heat to medium high.
5. Bring the broth to a boil, then reduce the heat to low and simmer for 15 minutes.
6. Add the pumpkin to the soup, and using an immersion blender, blend until creamy. If you do not have an immersion blender, transfer the soup in batches to a traditional blender and puree until creamy.
7. Stir in the almond milk until desired consistency is reached.
8. Continue cooking over low heat for 5 minutes.
9. Serve garnished with fresh parsley and walnuts.

Rustic Potato Soup

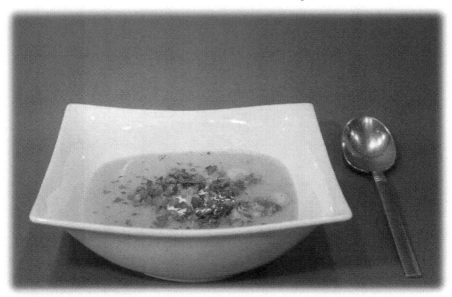

Servings: 6

Ingredients:

- ¼ lb. bacon, diced
- 6 medium sized potatoes, cut into cubes
- 2 cups carrots, diced
- 3 cups swiss chard, chopped
- ½ teaspoon salt
- ½ teaspoon black pepper
- 1 teaspoon dried thyme
- ¼ cup fresh parsley
- 2 tablespoons fresh chives
- 5 cups chicken or vegetable broth (FODMAP compliant)
- ½ cup fresh grated parmesan cheese
- ½ cup almond milk, or preferred FODMAP compliant milk alternative

Directions:

1. Place the bacon in a large soup pan or stock pot over medium high heat.
2. Cook the bacon, stirring frequently, until the bacon is browned and crisp.
3. Add the carrots, and cook while stirring for an additional 4-5 minutes.
4. Next, add in the swiss chard, potatoes, salt, black pepper, and thyme. Cook for 1-2 minutes.
5. Add in the broth and bring the liquid to a boil.
6. Once boiling, reduce the heat to low and simmer for 20 minutes, or until the potatoes and the carrots are tender.
7. Remove half of the soup, working in batches if necessary, and transfer it to a blender. Blend until creamy and then transfer it back into the pot with the rest of the soup.
8. Stir in the parsley, chives, parmesan cheese and almond milk.
9. Continue cooking over low heat for 5-10 minutes before serving.

Lemon Ginger Chicken and Rice Soup

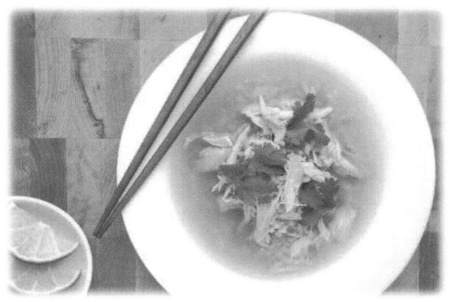

Servings: 4-6

Ingredients:

- 1 tablespoon olive oil
- 4 cups bok choy, shredded
- 2 tablespoons fresh grated ginger
- 1 teaspoon lemon zest
- 2 tablespoons soy sauce
- 2 tablespoons lemon juice
- 4-5 cups chicken broth (FODMAP compliant)
- 2 cups cooked, shredded chicken
- 2 cups cooked basmati rice
- 1 tablespoon fresh chives

Directions:

1. Heat the olive oil in a large soup pan or stock pot.

2. Once the oil is hot, add the bok choy, ginger and lemon zest. Cook, stirring frequently for 3-4 minutes.
3. Next, add in the lemon juice, soy sauce and chicken broth. Increase the heat to medium high and bring the liquid to a low boil.
4. Add in the shredded chicken and cooked rice. Reduce the heat to low and simmer for 10 minutes.
5. Serve garnished with fresh chives.

Curry Chicken Stew

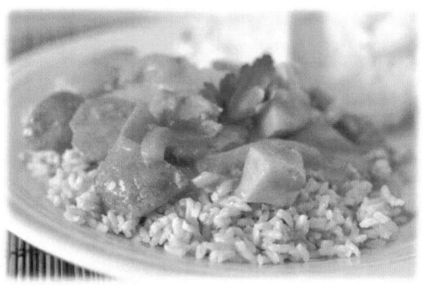

Servings: 4-6

Ingredients:

- 1 tablespoon olive oil
- 1 lb. boneless, skinless chicken breast, cubed
- 1 tablespoon curry powder (Check ingredients to make sure it doesn't contain added onion or garlic)
- 2 teaspoon garam masala (check ingredients to make sure it doesn't contain added onion or garlic)
- 1 teaspoon cumin
- ½ teaspoon salt
- ½ teaspoon black pepper
- 2 teaspoons fresh grated ginger
- 1 cup red bell pepper, chopped
- 4 cups potatoes, cubed
- 1 cup canned garbanzo beans, rinsed and drained
- 2 cups chicken broth (FODMAP compliant)
- 1 ½ cups preferred FODMAP compliant milk substitute

- 4 cups hot cooked basmati rice
- ¼ cup fresh mint, chopped

Directions:

1. Heat the olive oil in a deep skillet or soup pan.
2. Once the oil is hot, add in the chicken and season it with the curry powder, garam masala, cumin, salt and black pepper. Cook, stirring occasionally, until the chicken is browned.
3. Add in the ginger, red bell pepper and potatoes. Cook, stirring frequently for 5 minutes.
4. Next, add in the garbanzo beans and the chicken broth.
5. Increase the heat to medium high and bring the liquid to a low boil.
6. Reduce the heat to low and simmer for 15 minutes, stirring occasionally.
7. Add in the milk substitute and stir. Continue cooking until warmed through.
8. Serve the curry stew over hot rice, garnished with fresh mint.

Simple Beef Stew

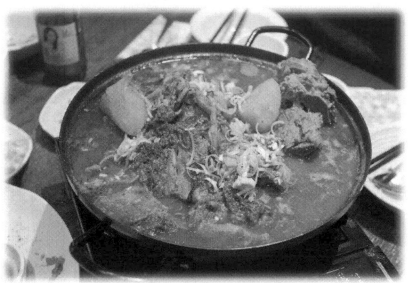

Servings: 6

Ingredients:

- 2 tablespoons arrowroot powder
- 1 teaspoon salt
- 1 teaspoon black pepper
- 1 ½ lb. stew meat
- 2 tablespoons butter
- ½ cup dry red wine (approved for cooking purposes)
- 2 cups potatoes, cubed
- 2 cups carrots, sliced
- 2 cups beef broth (FODMAP compliant)
- 1 tablespoon soy sauce
- 1 tablespoon tomato paste
- 1 bay leaf
- 1 teaspoon thyme
- 1 teaspoon oregano
- Cooked rice for serving

Directions:

1. In a bowl, combine the arrowroot powder with the salt and black pepper.
2. Add the stew meat to the flour and toss to lightly coat.
3. Heat the butter in a skillet over medium to medium high heat.
4. Add in the stew meat and cook, stirring frequently, until browned on all sides.
5. Add in the red wine and cook for 1-2 minutes until reduced. Use a spatula or wooden spoon to scrape up the browned bits from the skillet.
6. Remove the skillet from the heat and set aside.
7. Place the potatoes and the carrots in a slow cooker.
8. Add the stew meat, including any pan drippings into the slow cooker.
9. In a bowl, whisk together the beef broth, soy sauce and tomato paste.
10. Pour the liquid into the slow cooker and add the bay leaf, thyme and oregano.
11. Cover and cook on low for 8 hours.
12. Serve over cooked rice.

Scented Pork Stir-fry

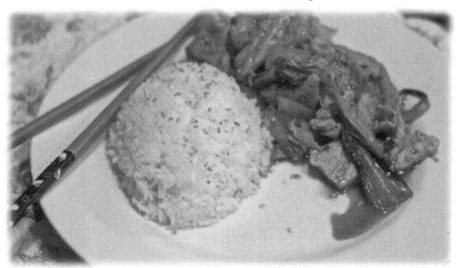

Servings: 4

Ingredients:

- 3 cups fresh green beans, trimmed
- 1 tablespoon olive oil
- 1 tablespoon sesame oil
- 1 lb. pork tenderloin, cut into thin strips
- ½ teaspoon salt
- ½ teaspoon black pepper
- 2 tablespoons soy sauce
- 1 tablespoon rice vinegar
- 1 teaspoon sugar
- 1 tablespoon fresh grated ginger
- 2 cups bok choy, shredded
- Hot, cooked rice for serving

Directions:

1. Bring a pot of lightly salted water to a boil.
2. Add in the green beans and cook them for 2-3 minutes.
3. Carefully remove the green beans from the boiling water and transfer them to a bowl of very cold water. Let sit for 1-2 minutes and drain.
4. Meanwhile, heat the olive oil and the sesame oil in a skillet over medium heat.
5. Add in the pork strips and season the meat with the salt and black pepper.
6. Cook, stirring frequently, just until the meat is browned.
7. While the meat is browning, whisk together the soy sauce, rice vinegar, sugar and ginger.
8. Add the bok choy to the skillet, along with sauce mixture. Cook for 1-2 minutes, before adding in the green beans.
9. Cook, stirring frequently, for an additional 2-3 minutes, or until the meat is cooked through.
10. Serve over hot cooked rice.

Chicken Fajita Plate

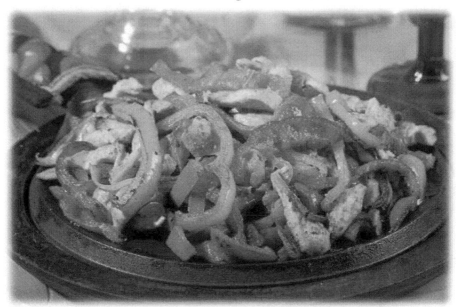

Servings: 4

Ingredients:

- 1 lb. boneless, skinless chicken breasts, sliced into strips
- 2 teaspoons lime juice
- ½ teaspoon salt
- ½ teaspoon black pepper
- 1 jalapeno pepper, seeded and minced
- 2 tablespoons olive oil
- 2 cups bell peppers, sliced
- 2 cups zucchini, sliced
- 4 cups baby spinach
- 3 cups cooked brown rice
- 1 teaspoon lime zest
- ¼ cup fresh cilantro

Directions:

1. Heat one tablespoon of the olive oil in a skillet over medium heat.
2. Sprinkle the chicken with the lime juice and season it with the salt and black pepper.
3. Place the chicken in the skillet and cook for 5 minutes, stirring occasionally.
4. Add the jalapenos, stir and cook for an additional 3-5 minutes, or until the chicken is cooked through.
5. Remove the chicken from the skillet and set aside.
6. Add the remaining oil to the skillet and add the bell peppers and zucchini. Cook, stirring frequently for several minutes until firm tender.
7. Add the baby spinach and cook until wilted.
8. Place the chicken alongside the vegetables on serving plates.
9. Place the rice in a bowl and add in the lime zest and cilantro.
10. Mix well and add to the plates to serve.

Sesame Beef and Rice

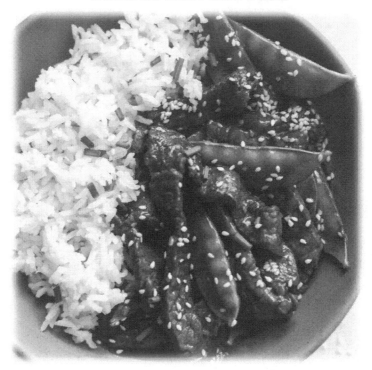

Servings: 4

Ingredients:

- 1 lb. beef steak, cut into thin strips
- ¼ cup soy sauce
- 1 tablespoon pure maple syrup
- 1 tablespoon lime juice
- 1 tablespoon sesame oil
- 2 teaspoons rice vinegar
- 12 ounces rice boodles
- 3 cups bok choy, chopped
- 3 cups fresh green beans, trimmed
- 1 tablespoon toasted sesame seeds
- 2 teaspoons olive oil

Directions:

1. In the bottom of a large bowl, combine the soy sauce, pure maple syrup, lime juice, sesame oil and rice vinegar. Whisk well.
2. Add the thinly sliced beef to the sauce and toss to coat. Set aside for 10-15 minutes.
3. Meanwhile, prepare the rice noodles according to package instructions, drain and set aside.
4. Heat the olive oil in the skillet over medium heat.
5. Add the green beans and sauté for 3-4 minutes, or until bright green and crisp tender. Add the bok choy and sauté an additional 2 minutes. Remove the vegetables from the skillet and set aside.
6. Add the beef, including any residual marinade into the skillet. Cook for 3-4 minutes, or until the meat is lightly browned.
7. Add the vegetables back into the skillet and cook until the vegetables are warmed through and the meat is cooked.
8. Add the noodles and toss.
9. Serve garnished with toasted sesame seeds.

Stuffed Peppers

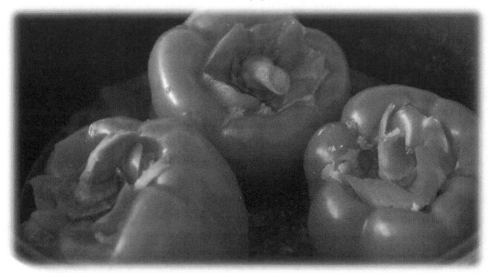

Servings: 4

Ingredients:

- 4 medium sizes bell peppers (color of choice)
- 1 lb. lean ground chicken
- ¼ cup soy sauce
- 4 cups baby spinach, chopped
- 1 cup zucchini, chopped
- 1 cup tomato, chopped
- ½ cup goat cheese
- ½ teaspoon salt
- ½ teaspoon black pepper
- 2 cups cooked quinoa
- 1 tablespoon olive oil

Directions:

1. Preheat the oven to 350°F and lightly oil and 8x8 inch baking dish.

2. Add the ground chicken to a skillet over medium heat.
3. Season the chicken with the soy sauce, salt and black pepper. Cook, stirring occasionally, until the chicken is cooked through.
4. While the chicken is cooking, cut the tops off the peppers and scoop out any seeds.
5. Place the cooked quinoa in a large bowl.
6. When the chicken is done, add it to the bowl with the quinoa.
7. Place the skillet back on the stove top and add the zucchini, baby spinach and tomatoes. Sauté for 4-5 minutes, then transfer to the bowl.
8. Add the goat cheese to the bowl and then stir all the ingredients together until well mixed.
9. Place the peppers in the baking dish.
10. Spoon the mixture into each of the pepper, placing any residual filling around the peppers in the baking dish.
11. Drizzle the peppers with olive oil and then cover the dish with aluminum foil.
12. Place the baking dish in the oven and bake for 25-30 minutes, or until the peppers are tender.

Cajun Steak with Twice Baked Potatoes

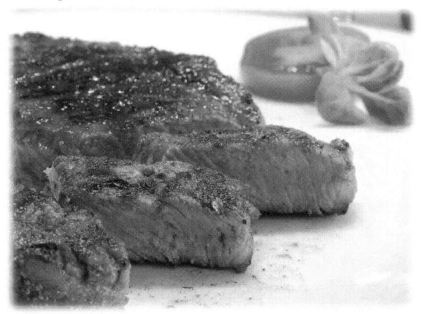

Servings: 4

Ingredients:
- 4 choice beef steaks, approximately 4 ounces each
- 1 tablespoon Cajun Rub (see recipe)
- 2 teaspoons olive oil
- 4 medium sized potatoes
- ½ teaspoon sea salt
- ½ cup cooked bacon, crumbled
- 2 tablespoons butter
- ½ cup goat cheese
- ½ cup lactose free milk
- 1 tablespoon chives
- ½ cup tomatoes, chopped

Directions:

1. Preheat the oven to 350°F.
2. Poke small holes in the potatoes and brush them with a little olive oil or butter and sprinkle them with the sea salt. Place them in the oven and bake for 45-50 minutes, or until tender. Remove them from the oven and set aside to cool enough to handle.
3. Once cool enough to handle, cut open the top of each potato and scoop out about ¾ of the insides and transfer them to a bowl.
4. To the bowl, add in the butter, goat cheese, and lactose free milk. Using a potato masher or electric mixer, mix until smooth.
5. Stir in the bacon, tomatoes and chives.
6. Spoon the mixture back into each of the potatoes, and then place them back in the 350°F oven for approximately 20 minutes, or until browned on top.
7. Meanwhile, preheat an indoor or outdoor grill over medium heat.
8. Brush the steaks with the olive oil and generously pat the Cajun Rub over the surface of the steaks.
9. Place the steaks on the grill and cook 5-7 minutes per side, depending on thickness and desired doneness.
10. Remove the steaks from the grill and let them rest at least 5 minutes before serving with the twice baked potatoes.

Swiss Stuffed Chicken

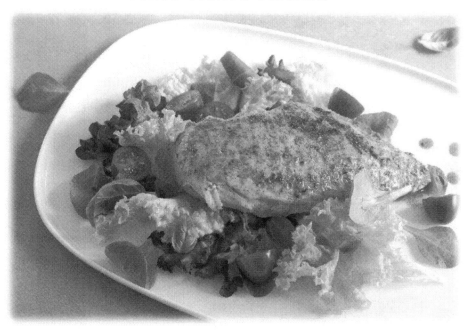

Servings: 4

Ingredients:

- 1 lb. boneless, skinless chicken breasts
- ½ teaspoon salt
- ½ teaspoon black pepper
- ¼ lb. bacon, diced
- 2 cups swiss chard, chopped
- 2 teaspoons coarse ground mustard
- 1 teaspoon pure maple syrup
- ¾ cup swiss cheese, shredded
- 1 cup cooked brown rice

Directions:

1. Preheat the oven to 375°F and lightly oil an 8x8 inch baking dish.

2. Place a cut along the side of each chicken breast, going about 2/3 of the way through. Season the chicken with the salt and black pepper and then set aside.
3. Place the bacon in a skillet over medium heat. Cook, stirring frequently, until the bacon is browned and crisp.
4. Using a slotted spoon, remove the bacon from the skillet and place it in a bowl with the cooked brown rice.
5. Next, add the swiss chard to the hot skillet with the bacon grease.
6. Add the mustard and maple syrup to the swiss chard and cook, stirring, until wilted. Transfer to the bowl with the bacon and rice.
7. Allow the ingredients in the bowl to cool slightly and then add in the swiss cheese.
8. Scoop equal amounts of the mixture into each of the chicken breasts, and then place them in the baking dish.
9. Place the baking dish in the oven and bake for 25-30 minutes, or until the chicken is cooked through.

Lemon Butter Shrimp over Vegetable Noodles

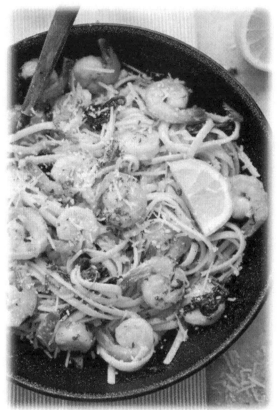

Servings: 4

Ingredients:

- 1 lb. shrimp, cleaned and deveined
- ¼ cup butter
- 1 tablespoon lemon juice
- 1 tablespoon capers
- ½ teaspoon salt
- ½ teaspoon black pepper
- 4 cups zucchini, spiral sliced into noodles

Directions:

1. Bring a lightly salted pot of water to a boil.
2. Add the zucchini spirals to the water and cook for 2-3 minutes.
3. Carefully remove the zucchini from the cooking water and transfer it to a bowl of ice water to stop the cooking. Let sit for 1-2 minutes before draining.
4. Heat the butter in a skillet over medium heat.
5. Sprinkle the shrimp with lemon juice and season it with the salt and black pepper.
6. Place the shrimp in the skillet with the butter, along with the capers.
7. Cook for 2-3 minutes per side, or until cooked through.
8. Add the zucchini noodles to the skillet and toss to coat in the warm butter.
9. Transfer to serving plates and enjoy.

Pineapple Shrimp Fajitas

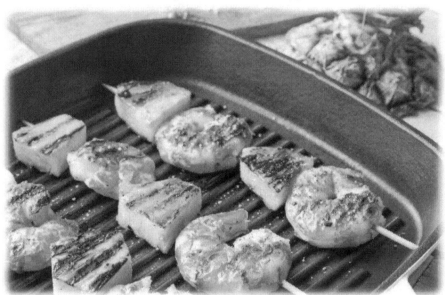

Servings: 4

Ingredients:

- 1 lb. shrimp, cleaned and deveined
- 2 tablespoons olive oil
- 2 tablespoons lime juice
- 1 tablespoon fresh chives
- 2 tablespoons fresh cilantro
- 1 cup pineapple chunks
- 2 cups red bell peppers, sliced
- 2 cups cooked brown rice
- 8-10 corn tortillas
- Metal or bamboo skewers

Directions:

1. In the bottom of a large bowl, whisk together the olive oil, lime juice, chives and cilantro.

2. Place the shrimp in the bowl, toss to coat and let sit for 5 minutes.
3. Preheat an indoor or outdoor grill over medium heat.
4. Place the shrimp on the skewers, alternating with pieces of pineapple.
5. Place the skewers on the grill and cook for 3-4 minutes per side, or until the shrimp is cooked through.
6. Meanwhile, spray a skillet with cooking spray and sauté the peppers over medium heat for 3-4 minutes, or until firm tender.
7. Remove the shrimp from the grill and serve with the sautéed peppers, cooked brown rice and corn tortillas.

Maple Salmon

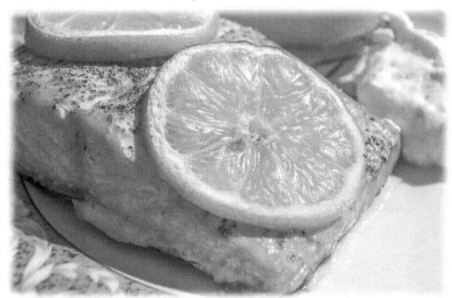

Servings: 4

Ingredients:

- 1 lb. salmon fillets
- 2 tablespoons soy sauce
- 2 tablespoons pure maple syrup
- 2 tablespoon fresh orange juice
- ½ teaspoon salt
- 1 teaspoon coarse ground black pepper

Directions:

1. Place the salmon fillets in a baking dish.
2. In a bowl, whisk together the soy sauce, maple syrup and orange juice.
3. Pour the marinade over the salmon, cover and refrigerate for up to two hours.

4. Preheat the oven to 350°F and line a baking sheet with aluminum foil.
5. Remove the salmon from the marinade and place it on the baking sheet.
6. Bake the salmon or 15-20 minutes, or until cooked through.

Salmon Patties with Caper Mayonnaise

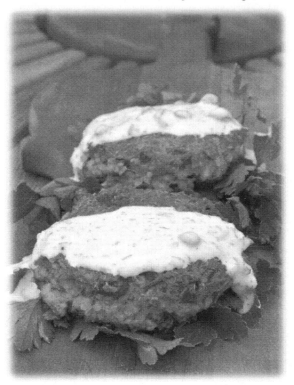

Servings: 4

Ingredients:

- 1 lb. cooked salmon, flaked
- 1 egg, beaten
- 2 tablespoons fresh dill
- 2 tablespoons fresh parsley
- ½ teaspoon salt
- ½ teaspoon black pepper
- 1 tablespoon olive oil
- ¼ cup mayonnaise (FODMAP compliant)
- 1 tablespoon lemon juice
- 1 tablespoon capers
- 2 teaspoons fresh chives

Directions:

1. In a bowl, combine the salmon, egg, dill, parsley, salt and black pepper. Mix well.
2. Brush a skillet with the olive oil and heat it over medium heat.
3. Using your hands, form eight equally sized patties and place them in the skillet.
4. Cook for approximately 4-5 minutes per side, or until nicely browned.
5. While the patties are cooking, quickly whisk together the mayonnaise, lemon juice, capers and chives.
6. Remove the salmon patties from the skillet and serve with the caper mayonnaise.

Fruits sauce

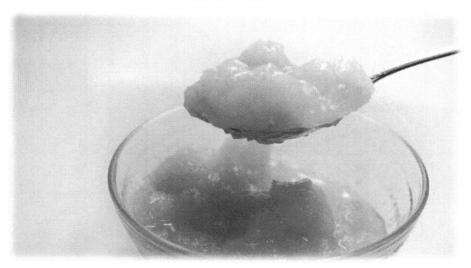

Servings: 4

Ingredients:

- 1 cup mango, cubed
- ½ cup pineapple juice
- 1 jalapeno pepper, seeded and minced
- 2 teaspoons miso paste

Directions:

1. Combine all the ingredients in a blender and blend until creamy.
2. Transfer the sauce to a saucepan over medium heat. Cook until it just starts to bubble.
3. Reduce the heat to low and simmer for 5 minutes before serving.

Southwest Fajita Dressing

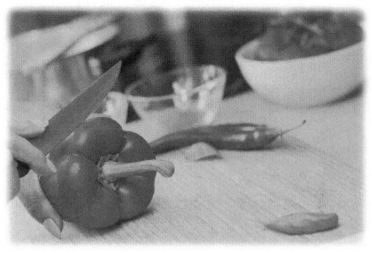

Servings: 6-8

Ingredients:

- ½ cup plain lactose free yogurt
- ¼ cup roasted red peppers
- 2 tablespoons olive oil
- ½ teaspoon paprika
- ½ teaspoon salt
- ½ teaspoon black pepper
- 1 tablespoon fresh chives
- 1 tablespoon fresh cilantro
- 2 teaspoons lime juice

Directions:

1. Combine all the ingredients in a blender and blend until smooth.
2. Store in a lidded container in the refrigerator. Mix well before using

Caper Dressing

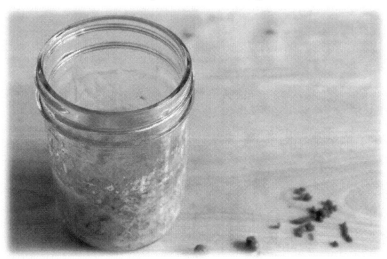

Servings: 6

Ingredients:

- ¼ cup olive oil
- ¼ cup champagne vinegar
- 2 teaspoons stone ground mustard
- 1 teaspoon lemon zest
- 1 tablespoon capers
- 2 teaspoons fresh chives
- ½ teaspoon salt
- ½ teaspoon black pepper

Directions:

1. Place all the ingredients in a bowl and whisk together until well blended.
2. Cover and store in the refrigerator. Mix well before using.

Raspberry Citrus Vinaigrette

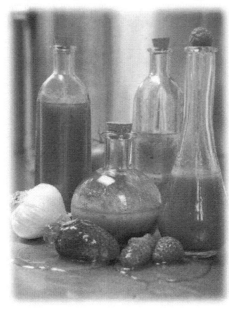

Servings: 8

Ingredients:

- ¼ cup olive oil
- 2 tablespoons lime juice
- ¼ cup orange juice
- ¼ cup fresh raspberries
- 1 teaspoon tarragon
- ½ teaspoon salt

Directions:

1. Combine all the ingredients in a blender and blend until smooth.
2. Transfer to a lidded container and keep in the refrigerator.
3. Mix well before using.

Cajun Rub

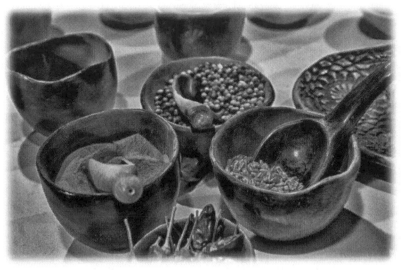

Servings: 4-6

Ingredients:

- 1 tablespoon paprika
- 1 teaspoon chili powder
- 2 teaspoons cumin
- 2 teaspoons mustard powder
- 1 teaspoon thyme
- 1 teaspoon coarse ground black pepper
- ½ teaspoon salt

Directions:

1. Place all ingredients in a lidded container, cover and shake.
2. Keep stored in an airtight container, away from moisture.

Desserts

Chocolate Covered Strawberries

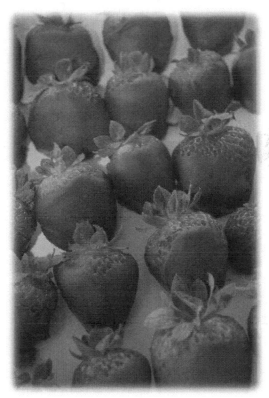

Serves: 4

Ingredients:
- 12 extra-large, ripe strawberries
- 1 cup dark chocolate pieces (at least 70% cocoa content)

Directions:
1. Line a baking sheet with parchment paper.

2. Place the chocolate pieces in the top part of a double boiler and melt over low heat while stirring.
3. Once the chocolate is melted, dip each of the strawberries into the chocolate.
4. Place the strawberries on the parchment paper.
5. Let sit for 15-20 minutes before serving.

Meyer Lemon Curd with Fresh Raspberries

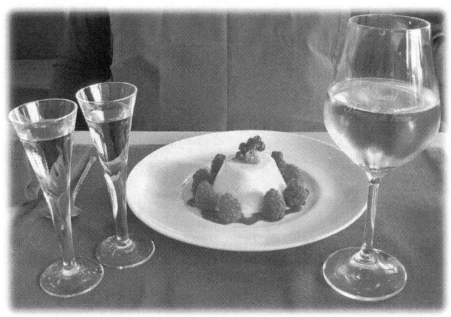

Serves: 4

Ingredients:
- 4 eggs
- 4 egg yolks
- 1 ½ cup sugar
- ½ cup butter
- ½ cup plus 2 tablespoons fresh squeezed Meyer lemon juice
- 1 tablespoon lemon zest
- 1 teaspoon pure vanilla extract
- 1 cup fresh raspberries
- 1 tablespoon fresh mint, chopped

Directions:

1. Combine the eggs, egg yolk, and sugar in a saucepan over low heat. Whisk continually until blended and warmed.
2. Add in the butter, Meyer lemon juice, lemon zest and vanilla extract. Continue whisking until the butter has completely melted in.
3. Increase the heat of the burner to medium and continue cooking and whisking until the curd thickens. This should take about 6-8 minutes.
4. Remove the curd from the heat, let it cool slightly then transfer it to a lidded container and place it in the refrigerator to cool.
5. Once cool, transfer to individual serving plates and garnish with fresh raspberries and mint.

Blueberry Banana Popsicle Blasts

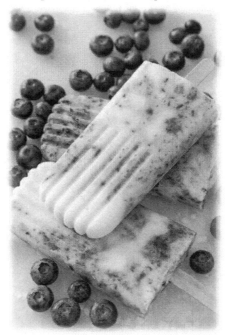

Serves: 4

Ingredients:

- 2 medium sized bananas, frozen and sliced
- 1 cup blueberries
- 1 cup fresh pineapple juice

Directions:

1. Place all the ingredients in a blender or food processor and blend until smooth.
2. Transfer the mixture to popsicle molds and freeze for at least 4 hours, or until set.

Cinnamon Butter Pecan Pralines

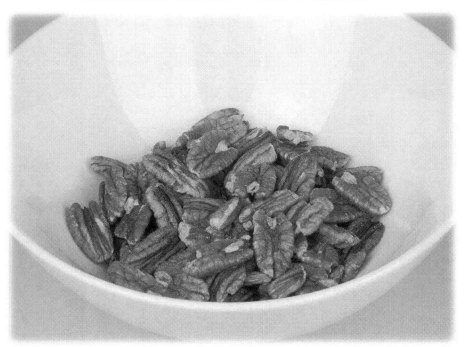

Serves: 6

Ingredients:

- ½ cup butter
- 1 ½ cups pecans, chopped
- 1 ½ cups white sugar
- ¾ cup brown sugar
- 1 teaspoon cinnamon
- 1 teaspoon pure vanilla extract
- ½ cup rice milk

Directions:

1. Line a baking sheet with aluminum foil or wax paper.
2. Combine all the ingredients in a saucepan over medium heat.

3. Cook, stirring frequently, for 10-15 minutes, or until the temperature on a candy thermometer reaches 240°F.
4. Take spoonfuls of the liquid mixture and make 12 equally sized circles on the prepared sheet.
5. Let sit until hardened before serving.

Low-FODMAP Trail Mix

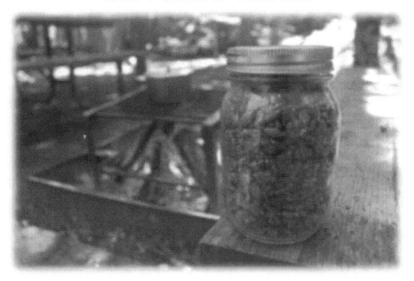

Serves: 4-6

Ingredients:
- 1 cup dried banana chips
- ½ cup walnuts
- ½ cup toasted pumpkin seeds
- ½ cup dark chocolate chips (at least 70% cocoa content)

Directions:

Combine all the ingredients and store in an airtight container.

Chive Dill Popcorn

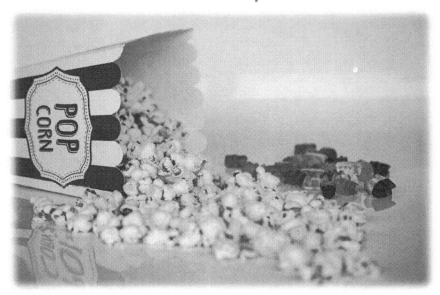

Serves: 4-6

Ingredients:

- 8 cups popped popcorn
- 1 tablespoon olive oil
- 1 tablespoon fresh chives
- 1 tablespoon fresh dill
- 1 tablespoon parmesan cheese

Directions:

1. Heat the olive oil chives and dill over low heat, just until warmed.
2. Drizzle the herbed oil over the popcorn and toss to coat.
3. Sprinkle with parmesan and toss before serving.

Cheese Stuffed Mini Tomatoes

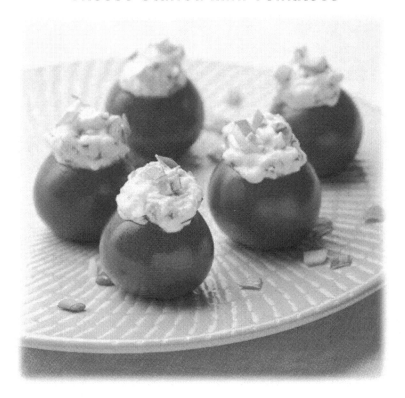

Serves: 4

Ingredients:

- 16 cherry tomatoes
- ½ cup goat cheese
- ¼ cup cooked bacon crumbles
- 1 tablespoon chives
- ½ teaspoon salt

Directions:

1. Slice off the very top of each of the tomatoes and carefully scoop out the insides. Place the tomato pulp in a bowl.

2. To the bowl with the tomato pulp, add in the goat cheese, bacon, chives and salt. Mix well.
3. Stuff the goat cheese mixture back into the tomatoes and serve.

Curried Roasted Chickpeas

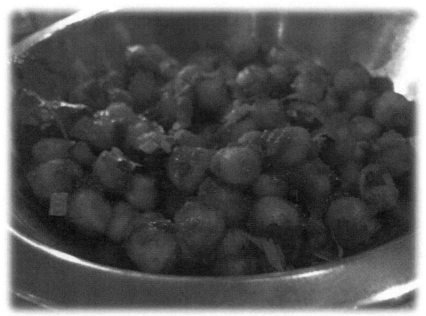

Serves: 4

Ingredients:

- 2 cups canned chickpeas
- 1 tablespoon olive oil
- 1 tablespoon apple cider vinegar
- 1 tablespoon curry powder (check ingredients for onion or garlic)
- ½ teaspoon salt

Directions:

1. Preheat the oven to 400°F and line a baking sheet with aluminum foil.
2. In a bowl, combine the olive oil, apple cider vinegar, curry powder and salt. Whisk together.
3. Add the chickpeas to the bowl and toss to coat.

4. Spread the chickpeas out on the baking sheet.
5. Place the baking sheet in the oven and bake for 50-60 minutes, stirring every 15 minutes, until golden brown.
6. Remove from the oven and let cool before serving.

Conclusion

Nobody wants to live with the pain and discomfort of IBS and other digestive disorders, and the truth is that no one should have to. While the low-FODMAP diet isn't a cure for digestive and intestinal disease, it is a method of effectively managing your symptoms and improving your quality of life. IBS, and similar conditions, are different from many other chronic diseases that you can treat with medication. Because IBS can be so individualized, it is difficult to fully treat. Instead, you look towards learning what causes your symptoms and learning how to manage them. This is what this book has been intended to do.

Going through a FODMAP elimination plan is a journey of self-discovery. Of course, the main goal is to discover some of the foods that might be making your symptoms worse, but chances are you will discover more about yourself during the process. You will learn more about your body, how it responds to food and how you emotionally connect with food.

Remember that the low-FODMAP plan is not intended to be a long-term lifestyle. If you choose to forever eliminate these foods, you will be missing out not only on nutritional value, but also providing your gut with food for the good bacteria that helps to keep you healthy. Stick with the full plan for only 4 weeks, and then decide, preferably during a discussion with your doctor, which foods to include, which to eliminate and which to enjoy in moderation for your typical daily diet.

All types of new dietary plans take some getting used to and a little bit of willpower, but remember, this plan is not meant to restrict your calories or the pleasure you gain from sharing food with friends or family. It is meant instead to help you enjoy food without painful side effects. Keep this in mind during those times when temptation starts to pop in. The recipes included in this book have been designed to be simple and delicious. My hope is that this will help you keep on track with your dietary goals.

Finally, embrace the change that you are making with your body. You are taking charge of your health and regaining control of your life, both of which are truly wonderful things.

Dear Reader,
Thank you for buying and reading my book!
If you like it, please, leave a review. It is important for me and my future books.
Just scan this code and you can leave a review

Or just type this link – https://www.amazon.com/review/create-review?ie=UTF8&asin=B075FD1TLT#

Made in the USA
San Bernardino, CA
11 December 2017